JO MAY

A Bike at Large

To Jan

Thanks for all the wonderful years.
It's you who's made these adventures sing...

Give a man a fish and feed him for a day.

Teach a man to fish and feed him for a lifetime.

Teach a man to cycle and he will realize fishing is boring and stupid.

Desmond Tutu

Contents

I

Part One

A new world on two wheels

1

Starting gait....

At the end of this book, I've written an introduction. The final chapter, which I've called *The Vault*, explains why I have revisited the world of bicycles. It also tells you why I partake of manic exercise in general. But that's all at the end because I don't really want to focus on it. I'd rather share some more pleasant bits with you. If you want to have an idea about the why, go and have a look. The final chapter is optional. A peculiar set-up, but there we are. What it boils down to is that you can ignore the introduction. If I was in your shoes I probably would, largely because I'm a man and we men tend to ignore important things and get straight to essential things like beer or football, or sharing things with my Mrs - who, as I said in the dedication, makes our adventures sing.

What I will do in the following pages is tell you about some of the daft things that happened while cycling, as well as how I chose my e-bike then gingerly learned to cope with it - which did result in the odd bandage! I'll also explain how I cycled into a big hole in the road in Holland on my very smart €40 bicycle - an embarrassing and uncomfortable episode. I hadn't seen the hole because I was hurtling along, head down, 200-meters from the finish line and glory in the Tour de France. I was in that state of Nirvana achieved by an elite athlete where man and machine are lost in a subconscious other world.

I have met some quirky people (I seem to attract them actually); recently, for example, I encountered Mr Slightly Ratty in Cumbria, a man constantly on the brink of a temper explosion. I'll tell you some of the amazing places I've cycled round, like Verdun - the scene of the most brutal of battles. Remembering things like this is grounding; it gives a perspective to everything else; it makes the good times all the sweeter; it makes me more tolerant of people.

I have friends and acquaintances who have mental health struggles, so I am aware that anybody I encounter could be one ill-judged comment from jumping off a bridge - stark but true. When I think of the headstones of those who have gone, I'm less tolerant of all the fripperies that fill our lives, the bling and tat that has replaced the really important things, like community, respect, tolerance and the wonderful natural world we have around us, too often taken for granted.

This is not an A to B directory, nor is it a tourist information guide. Any information you may garner regarding the routes to take or the nature of places I describe is incidental. These are my impressions, viewed through my eyes, which are red/green colour blind - so what I see as red may not be what you see as red.

Those who have read my three boating books in the **At Large** series will know my style. In truth, some people get ratty with me for not being a tourist guide. Tough luck - there are plenty of those already. One reviewer suggested I include maps in the boating books, and my 'oversight' cost me at least one star. I don't have a right of reply to reviews, which is probably a good job really. One woman, who gave me a real stinker, would probably not have been appeased had I been able to suggest she seek psychiatric assistance. Lots of people have said lovely things but it's the one bad one that sticks in the mind - 'keeps me honest' as the saying goes.

It's like having a perfect physiognomy but being lumbered with a big red wart on one's nose. In my case a lone red wart would be a delight, considering all the other anomalies that make up the badly wrapped package that is me. I'm short and dumpy, so I never look entirely comfortable no matter how much I spend on clothes - which is perhaps why I fitted into the boating existence so well, because it was almost a prerequisite to look like a vagrant. My physique is probably not best suited to Lycra. Fleshy bits tend to squeeze out, which is why I wear a top layer. On one occasion I sported jogging bottoms; though they have never been jogging, they did get me in a pickle. I'll explain that episode in due course.

Yes, I've loved cycling over the years. Like many people, I have cycled since I was a child. Once you've conquered that first ten yards without a break, physical or temporal, you're off and away for ever. Adults cycle to the shop, or work, to keep fit or just for fun. For a child, the bicycle is a conduit between all sorts of misdemeanors; often a means of escape, from homework perhaps, or the door you've just knocked on. There's freedom for a youngster, an exciting way to have fun with your mates, and a great way to keep fit and develop young physiques.

You're fearless in your youth. Falling off isn't an issue - you just get back on again. Speed is of no concern, the faster the better. I remember whoopin' and hollerin' with my mate hurtling down a hill, screaming with delight, till he fell off and lost his kneecap. Horrid that. But when the plaster came off he got straight back on his bike again. The nastiness of his injury was locked in his chest of drawers of times past, so the present was free of worry. Back up the hill, down again. More hollerin.' I broke both my arms once, at the same time. As a thirteen-year-old I was knocked off my bike and landed head-first. I had my arms over my head for protection. I had my judo coach to thank for teaching me that instinctive self-preservation manoeuvre. My arms took the brunt ... and crunch. They weren't bad breaks, but bad enough for plaster casts from elbow to wrists (which made certain bodily tasks awkward). But even before the plasters came off I was riding again.

That was nearly fifty years ago. It was a cream-coloured VW Beetle driven by Mr Carson that nearly brought a premature end to my cycling, and my life. The car windows were steamed up on a murky November morning and he came out of a junction straight into the side of me. I've never forgotten that painful lesson. Never, ever, trust a car driver. I was actually more bothered about my bike than my body. I was on the way back from the cycle shop where my Raleigh Olympus (yes, I remember - red, black and silver it was) had just been serviced. It was going like a dream before it got rearranged under the Beetle. But as a youngster, I was back on track in no time. Resilience. That's what you have as a youth. Bounce back. (Perhaps that historic episode is why I, subconsciously, liken myself to a corpulent beetle while shuffling around the highways and byways.)

Then the years rumble on and you appreciate the dangers involved. Particularly on the main roads, as they have got busier and busier. Back in Mr Carson's day there were much fewer cars. In fact, he and I were unlucky in coming together like we did. Like the Titanic and her iceberg, it was largely fate - with some incompetence thrown in. The standard of driving has deteriorated as people get more fraught, silently cocooned in ever-faster cars. I can't say that cycling on main roads is a pleasure; it's a means to getting somewhere safe and fun. After all, you don't get many second chances when bike and car collide.

I can't remember a time when I was without a bike, whether living on land or on a boat. My way to avoid the worst of the traffic has always been to go out early. Formerly a baker, I developed an early bird habit and have never lost it. Early is my time of day, a magical time when there's nobody else to wreck it. It's just me and the wildlife and the odd milkman. We lived in rural Shropshire for a while where the roads were quiet. While boating we had the towpaths, which were ideal. Not only that, while we were afloat our bikes were our only form of transport. It was a pretty healthy lifestyle. Except, idiotically, I was a smoker. That habit got me in big trouble. I've explained a bit about that in *The Vault.*

On the continent, particularly rural France, there are many hundreds of miles of quiet roads. When you're poddling along at ten miles per hour, you realize just how vast France is. Through endless forests of oak where the hiss of the silence can be deafening. I'd ride with rumbling tractors for company as farmers tended enormous tracts of farmland. I'd pass through sleepy villages with dozy dogs, tiny places apparently abandoned to the past. Holland is geared for cyclists. The bicycle is king and woe betide any car driver who dents a cyclist. There are dedicated cycle paths running parallel to many roads so it's a safe and enjoyable way to get around. Families, sometimes four to a bike (when you include a toddler-trailer tacked on the back), share cycleways with Lycra-clad speedsters and shoppers of all ages, panniers laden with gehaktballen (meatballs) or snert (explosive pea and ham soup).

I had a brief period where I didn't cycle. During that time I got porkier and less fit, till I decided to try and pull myself together. My enthusiasm is rediscovered because my e-bike has allowed me to return to a time when I could cycle just about anywhere. To a degree, my limit these days is dictated by battery life. So here follows some tales. They'll be largely focused on cycling but also a bit of walking. Both activities have enabled me to do my best for myself, a self I'd previously neglected and stupidly taken for granted.

2

And We're Off! (Well, sort of...)

I've just paid for an electric bike. It's a battery-assisted e-bike or bat bike. *Paid for,* note. I can't have it yet because of supply problems. Seems everybody wants to cycle during the Covid pandemic. Six weeks the wait. I'm going to call it Columbanus. Why? Because Columbanus is the patron saint of motorcyclists. I will have a cycle with a motor, so it's near enough. Plus, it sounds rather like *'numb anus'* - which sort of sums it up.

The make and model is *Lectro Peak* - a brand nobody has heard of, apart from the shop where I bought it and the Korean bloke who stuck on the go-faster decals. It has one rechargeable battery and two engines. The main engine is in the back wheel, powered by the battery. This appears very efficient. The secondary engine is a double piston arrangement attached to my buttocks, otherwise known as legs. The latter is a vintage model and is less efficient. Truth be known, it's in need of a re-bore. Hardly surprising, really - it's had a lot to put up with, including lugging an increasingly portly top half around the northern hemisphere for a long time.

So, why an e-bike? Well, I thought I'd like to get back into cycling after a spell out of the game. But it didn't get off to the most auspicious start ... my first practice cycle for nearly five years was a disappointing affair. I borrowed a mountain bike from my stepdaughter. It's an uncomfortable black thing that doesn't go very fast despite having lots of gears. By way of example, while cycling a local canal towpath, negotiating a slight incline (and I mean slight) I was overtaken by a jogger. Yes, a jogger. Not a runner, a jogger. To compound the ignominy, our jogger, to put it tactfully, was carrying a little weight.

Oh dear ...

Rather embarrassed, I realized I needed help so raided my wife's piggy bank and bought the e-bike. I promised her I'd be able to get even further out of her hair, which seemed to swing it. I love being out and about, so have to find a way to explore without compromising my self-esteem. On more than one occasion while mounting an incline on my stepdaughter's duff machine, the old legs have temporarily given up. This meant I came to a grinding halt so I had to pretend to be taking a photo of something interesting in a hedge. (Notice I don't refer to them as hills - they don't come into that category; they are inclines similar in length and steepness to those you find outside the chemist, where I go for my buttock salve.) I decided an e-bike was the answer. Whatever, this new beast has to be an improvement on being bettered by a porky jogger.

What am I really doing? Am I searching for eternal youth on this great e-bicycle adventure? No. It's more fundamental than that. Frankly, I'm trying to stay out of my eternal hole in the ground. A pressing matter upon which I must take decisive action, pretty swiftly. I'm a chap of 61. If you've come across my photo you'll see, despite the wonders of Photoshop, I have dutifully cultivated a weathered exterior. If you think what's on view is bad, the rest, below the surface, is even more knackered! I have the odd self-induced health issue, dodgy arteries mainly. Most people 'of an age' have something to fret about, so perhaps you'll empathize.

Right, as I said I've been a bit sneaky and put the 'introduction' at the end of the book. Peculiar I realize, but it's back there as a sort of reference point and to be read only if you want to. It's really a datum point for me to refer to as I lurch from pain to pleasure and back having relaunched my cycling endeavours. I'll find out soon enough how much progress I'm making.

Here, within the following pages, I will chronicle my latest attempt to behave like an athlete. My inadequacies will be laid bare in all their dysfunctional glory. While compiling this compendium my memory coughed up some long-forgotten snippets from cycling days gone by.

Actually, as far as this book's concerned, I was spurred into action by a friend of mine, a guy a decade older than me. He cycled (non-electric) the length of the British Isles in two weeks. Now that's a thousand miles, give or take a few yards, and a fabulous achievement that deserves to be trumpeted. I sponsored him. Realizing that my initial generosity 'knew bounds,' I doubled it to 2p per mile, split between 1p for the downhill bits and 3p for the climbs. Well done, Kevin Blick. What he wouldn't have been able to do as much as he would have liked, because of time restraints, is stop and smell the roses along the way (to paraphrase golfer Walter Hagen). Here, I have time to smell the roses. Most of them are fragrant and pretty, and the odd one is malodourous and pretty nasty.

So, if you're ready … here we go.

3

Free Wheels?

How did I plan my new purchase? My search began on the Internet, of course. I could plan my cycling future with no physical effort whatsoever. E-bikes are big business - the web is awash with them (or was - as I write, it's August 2020). So popular has biking become throughout the lockdown that many models are 'out of stock.' The photos are still there, but they have become e-ghosts -a tantalizing glimpse of what we can't have.

I'll readily admit that it was all new to me. I discovered that new ones cost from £500 up to £10k or more. The majority seem to be in the middle / lower price bracket, say £1,000 to £2,500. There are crank-driven or hub-driven models with a choice of different size motors. A variety of battery sizes give different power and/or range. There are road bikes, mountain bikes and hybrids. There's also a choice of frame (step-through / crossbar) and wheel sizes and you can even have one that folds up to pop in the boot of the car.

I learned there are basically two locations for the motor - in the crank (the central section low down between the pedals) or in the wheel hubs. It's more commonly at the rear but occasionally the front. The crank models are for more serious (fitter, more adventurous) bikers and are much more expensive. So, hub it is. A *'pedal assist'* e-bike is where the rider pedals normally and the battery and motor combine to help you, adding to your own effort by varying degrees dependent on the setting you choose. Pedal assist means you can travel not only further and faster but also tackle hills without trouble. It's this last bit that really interests me because it's where I'm really struggling. I can walk, but barely run. On a normal bike I'm just about OK on the flat but no good on an incline. I have this recurring porky jogger dream. I need electric therapy.

Now, the battery. We had lots of batteries when we had a boat - different types for different jobs; deep cycle leisure batteries are for the domestic supply, lights, pumps, etc., and those with high cranking power are for engine starting (like we have in our cars - those with an internal combustion engine, anyway). Batteries were the heartbeat of our boats when we were not connected to mains power, and capacity and output had to be married to our requirements. I guess it is the same with a bike. It's a relationship between volts, amps and watts, one that I'm not over-confident with. Matching battery with motor is important, so I leave that to someone else.

Armed with a few ideas and my new-found knowledge, I decide I need a face-to-face consult. There's a bike shop local to where I live, about 250 yards away - that's very nearly walking distance! It's called *The Ride Stuff* and the proprietor is Paul. Turns out he's a helpful lad, and a good man with whom to have a consult. The shop is at the top of an external flight of stairs, the metal fire-escape type. This is not ideal for me. By the time I lug my stomach to the summit I am in need of an isotonic drink. Fifteen feet up is not ideal for a bike shop either, you'd have thought, but there we are. Perhaps the rent is cheap. Actually there's a snooker club downstairs so I doubt the floor would stand the weight of a dozen or so tables if they swapped it around.

My initial thought had been a hybrid. I'd ruled out a road bike (droopy handlebars and knife-thin wheels) because I wanted to cycle on the canal towpaths and rougher tracks on the moors. In the end, Paul persuades me to get a mountain bike because they rule nothing out - roads, hills, tracks, wherever. I agree. He shows me one on the computer that has been selling well and has good feedback. They have been selling so well he hasn't got any in stock. In fact, there is nothing I can have immediately; as I've said, I had to wait about six weeks. That is slightly disappointing, but a shorter wait than other places - and I am supporting a local shop. Independent shopkeepers have had a tough enough time recently. I'd like to see our town, like many others, come out of the current mess at least as healthy as before. Besides, I can use the intervening time to build up my massive (-ly disappointing) thigh muscles while riding my daughter's inadequate boneshaker.

4

Reading myself fit

Ongoing preparations for the relaunch of my cycling odyssey include reading, something else that also requires very little physical effort. Specifically, a magazine - a birthday present from my wife. Not the whole birthday present you understand, just part of it. The socks (a present from the dog) will doubtless come in handy too! And the handkerchief. I'm being rude - the main present was a pair of binoculars, and crackers they are too. I look forward to benefiting from them if I ever climb a hill.

I'm still in the research phase of *'Operation Pork.'* I'm excitedly awaiting delivery of my e-bike. But I'm putting pen to paper following my miserable struggles on my step-daughter's useless bike. I've come to hate that infernal machine. What it boils down to is that I'm full of enthusiasm but have taken a knock to the self-esteem. Therefore I'm reading the magazine to try and convince myself I'm a proper cyclist, or will be when I get my battery charged. I'm psyching myself up, getting my head (which is frequently somewhere else) in gear.

I am idly flicking through my mag and get that unmistakable whiff of quality, the odour of top-notch, glossy magazine. Preparations for *'Operation Pork'* include diet, so I'm reading while lunching on smoked salmon (responsibly sourced - from Lidl) with scrambled eggs (free range – also from Lidl) on carbohydrate-free buttered toast (£15 for 3 keto loaves from a company in Hertfordshire, delivery to my fridge included).

I soon became quite depressed. Not with the lunch - my protein fest is ideal preparation for body and brain to tackle the next few hours. No, it's the magazine content. I've had the magazine a while and before I picked it up today it had been sitting on the coffee table hidden away under an old copy of *Lancashire Life*. I had had a brief look through on my birthday, but nothing had really registered. Being a birthday, I was just too excited to concentrate properly. I was more bothered about playing with my other presents, like my dog socks. In fact, I couldn't have even told you what it was called, '*Cycling....* *er, something.*' *Cycling Plus*, that's the name. Of course it is.

But now I'm eager to learn and take advice, so I concentrate. First impressions of the mag are OK. In fact, more than OK. There are crisp photos of impossibly fit people on gleaming machines in captivating settings. It is when I dig a little deeper that I become rather, er, overawed. The first article I flicked to, quite by chance, is by a professor who looks decades older than me. I'm not even guaranteed to live another decade, so seeing this chap in bloom at that age is sobering. If I've grasped it right, he's 85. I'm 61 with one or two health issues. That basically means that I ruined my health and am now playing catch-up, trying to keep the word 'still' before 'alive,' as opposed to 'no longer.' I put my envy aside and decide good on the prof. for continuing his active existence and giving me something to aim for. He's discussing age and what level of fitness one should expect at various milestones. I ignore the technical bits because I don't really fit into an age/fitness box. I am where I am, end of story.

Another article, that flops open as I'm nearing the end of my salmon, details the test of an Italian bike. The man testing it looks fit as a fiddle and the machine is a multi-thousand pound budget-buster (my budget, anyway). The location is indecipherable because the photos are shot with a blurred background. This has the effect of highlighting in sharp focus man and bike, which are the important things after all. This technique also enhances the effect of speed and endeavour. But, wherever he is, it's obvious he's making splendid progress. As I write, we're in lockdown so I can only dream about progressing further than the end of our avenue. Plus, my bike hasn't arrived yet and I'm a stone over ideal, so at this stage it's difficult to compare me with a god in a magazine. I need to sort myself out here or my cycling ambitions will founder before they get cracking. I have to change the mindset, select the right gear for the climb ...

Then, an epiphany. I realize that they only feature the crème de la crème in these mags, both people and hardware. They certainly wouldn't feature a blob like me on a 40-euro junker. No, mere mortals are simply not glossy enough for silken pages. The thing I have to do is drag them down a few notches, nearer to my (modest) level. I use my prodigious imagination to visualise the bike tester to be younger than me, but looking much older. I chortle to myself as I imagine his flat stomach being held together by an industrial gusset and chuckle louder at the image of his Lycra shorts that include plastic inserts to make it look like he has rippling Cavendish thighs. The bike itself would have been plucked from a scrap heap and re-sprayed by a back-street paint specialist in Nuneaton, at little cost. The photo would have been taken in front of a large mural in a studio in Rochdale. There's nothing intrinsically wrong with Rochdale, I might add - it just happens to be the nearest horrid place to where I live. Now I think about it, the best photos of Rochdale are blurred. There. That feels better. Not so bloody clever now are you, old chap on your fancy Italian machine?! It is a lovely-looking bike, though (sob).

I still have to get (psychologically) past more derring-do articles, like cycling right round a Scottish island, and the eye-catching adverts. For example, there was a pair of sunglasses that cost more than my brother's pedigree dog- which wasn't cheap. Perhaps not a bad analogy really. Pedigree dogs can be less hardy than mutts of indeterminate origin - overly fine breeding can make them susceptible to all manner of expensive ailments. So, would a finely-tuned bicycle really suit me, an athlete who not only carries a touch of extra ballast but who also lives in the Lancashire Pennines where all sorts of unpleasant illnesses lurk in the soot-stained infrastructure?

I also have to get over the price of things. The featured bike, mentioned above, cost four thousand pounds **more** than the £1,400 I've just balked at paying for mine – and this one hasn't even got an engine! I need to investigate. I'm sure that technically things have moved on while I have been slobbing around the continent on my €40 potterer.

The first thing I note is that it has an 'Elite' Bottle Cage. That's the thing that holds your water bottle, or isotonic pick-me-up or, in my case, red wine (case, huh!). 'Elite' with a capital letter, note, so that means it's a brand or manufacturer rather than an adjective. I wonder what else they make. I Google. Cycle trainers are one thing - apparatus that allows you to train in your coal shed during poor weather. They also make the bottles that go in their cages. Elite. I'll have to look out for that - the name sort of suits my athletic aura (!). Had it been called a 'Globule' Bottle Cage, I wouldn't have given it a second glance. Actually, now I think about it, the bottle cage was included in the price - on my bike it was an added extra, along with numerous other bits and pieces that the manufacturer thoughtfully left off!

The Italian bike weighs in at a fraction over 8kg. Mine is about 25. To demonstrate just how I'm trying to turn my gloomy outlook around, I look at it this way: the superbike will set you back nearly £700 a kilo. Mine, £56. There, I knew I'd got a bargain. It's thinking like this that's got me where I am today! (Actually today it's raining, so I'm writing while day-dreaming of the open road and potholes. As part of the regime I'm drinking de-caf coffee, ethically sourced - from Lidl. Yes, that's where I am today. On my glutes.)

It's obvious I'm struggling a bit, isn't it? I'm in a bit of turmoil. There's a section talking about the wheels where I only understand about one word in seven. The wheel section runs appropriately into the tyre section, which proves to be another delve into the realms of mysticism, including (to me) hugely high pressures and graphene. I doubt graphene featured on my Raleigh Olympus. I'm sure that the Italian job is a superb piece of kit; it certainly looks it. Seriously, I'm not taking the piss - I am genuinely flummoxed by the world of modern cycling.

I flick back to the beginning of the magazine and I note with some interest that the editor's introduction has a photo of him looking a touch porky. He readily admits that lockdown has meant severely restricted exercise, so he actually looks quite 'normal' - like me, in fact. I detect a chink of light within this silken mag, a whiff of honesty - which is never a bad thing. In fact, I read through it and thoroughly enjoy it. I'm a bit frustrated I physically can't do some of the suggested rides and wish I could afford all the latest gadgetry, because I am absolutely convinced that I'd be a world-beater with more impressive tackle.

I'm also disappointed that, unless I have a late career change, I'll never be eligible to be a member of the PPCC. I have to smile at this. It's a cycling club formed in 2016 (I think) but was 'unaffiliated' by British Cycling a year or two later. British Cycling is the governing body for cycle sport in Britain. They found out that PPCC stood for Porn Pedallers Cycling Club. Apparently, it's an accurate description because all its members are associated with the 'adult film entertainment industry.' Brilliant!

British Cycling endorse the mantra that 'Cycling Is For Everyone.' 'Except us', say the beleaguered Porn Pedallers. Last I heard, talks are ongoing to find a way for PPCC to rejoin the fold, but it appears the wheels of cycling justice turn slowly indeed. Needless to say, they got huge publicity from this travesty and have not looked back since. Good for them!

5

Got It! (But there's an early niggle ...)

I 'm rooting around in the kitchen cupboard looking for a bandage. I've got a nasty scrape on my hand (sigh). Let me explain ... I'd sent my friend Nigel a photo of Columbanus. He's a year or two older than me and recently moved to Spain where cycling weather is more old-git friendly. He is also a very experienced cyclist, despite having had (at least) one ankle fused. He's a useful man to know. When he buys something he does his research, so this is not the first time I've sought his advice (solar panels and motor car were others). Of course, I don't have to accept his advice.

'Don't like those extra-wide handlebars,' he emailed back.

'You're a dinosaur,' I tell him, from the safety of another country. 'This is how they are in the modern era.'

My bike is pretty heavy. About 25 kilos. That's a bag and a quarter of smokeless fuel! I know - I used to lug plenty of those onto the boat. A normal mountain bike is around 12 or 13 kilos, so it's the battery and motor on an e-bike that account for the extra weight. Perch me on top, a lump who is a 'conservative' stone over ideal, and the whole combo is quite weighty. It's got disc brakes, which are new to me, so should be able to stop OK, but I will have to be wary of those fragile canal bridges. Don't want to end up collapsing one and ending up in the cut.

Paul the bike shop guy watches me carefully as he talks me through the bike's features (and takes my money). He sees me slowly regain some sort of equilibrium having climbed the stairs to his first-floor shop. By the time he's finished his spiel my colour is near normal. Despite this he offers to carry my bike down the stairs. An act of benevolence? Good customer relations? Or the fact that he doesn't want the inconvenience of a new customer expiring on his premises? He asks if I can manage to carry the battery charger and lead. He doesn't smirk so I can only think he's being courteous rather than scoffing.

Time for a test run. I receive concise instructions and set off from the bottom of the fire escape under Paul's watchful eye. I am to test out the gear change in various power modes while trundling round the car park, then return to base camp. The car park is quite large; it services a number of businesses, including the snooker club. I'd honed my physique in a similar club in times past, waggling one arm about and drinking stout. There's a lot of bending over playing snooker, you know.

Anyhow, as I set off I misjudge the width of the bike and scrape my hand against the stone wall. The bike's quite wide you see, compared to some, and … well, best not mention this little mishap to Nigel. Barely a niggle, really - I'll keep it to myself.

If you remember, part of the reason I've bought an electric thing is to preserve my self-esteem. I resolve to practice without an audience. Right, off we go. It's half a mile home but the battery monitor is showing red. Why does red always stand out more than green? The monitor has 4 LED lights and it's pretty obvious what the red one means. With battery charger and lead in an orange Sainsbury's shopping bag I wobble away. There are four power settings ranging from 0 to 4. Zero is leg power only, which is not advised for an old wreck like me, particularly because of the pre-mentioned weight issue (me and the bike). Setting 4 is maximum warp speed, for steep hills and lightning acceleration.

'Bring it back in six weeks for a free check-over,' Paul says as I leave. I wave over my shoulder as I set off down Sutcliffe Street, pedalling like mad to build up a head of steam in case the battery runs out. Thankfully it lasts fine and I get home without further injury.

Three fifths of a mile recorded on my e-tachometer. Only one minor injury for the accident book. Fitness report: no noticeable improvement.

I park the bike in the garage and dash to the kitchen to bandage my hand then return to the garage to plug in the charger. I'm back ten minutes later to make sure everything is OK, in particular that the Taiwanese battery charger hasn't gone up in flames, taking the garage with it. I've always been a bit wary of leaving things plugged in.

Then, to my surprise, I notice that the front tyre is flat. I wonder whether this will happen every time I plug it in. Of course, I haven't got any repair tackle. I ring the bike shop and speak to Paul's assistant, asking him if they have a puncture repair outfit he can throw in as part of my purchase or, at worst, buy as an extra. He is a bit brusque, frankly, and tells me I should just buy a replacement inner tube. I put the phone down wondering if he thinks I am made of money. Out of spite I order a repair kit and some tyre levers from Halfords, a major bicycle (and motor car parts) retailer. Click and collect same day - good service.

I look over my new steed and realize I need a few more things which haven't come as standard, despite paying a hefty amount for the bike. I am short of a pump, bell, water-bottle holder (I'll see if I can find an 'Elite' one), security lock, small bag to Velcro to the crossbar, gloves, rear light, mud-guards and a helmet. So by the time I finish my 'Lifestyle Investment' has set me back in excess of £1,400. Then, of course, there is clothing! I can't hurtle about on an expensive piece of equipment looking like a tramp (like I usually do). No, I need something to reflect my cycleworthyness. Nearly £1,500 now! But...

By calling Columbanus a Lifestyle Investment I've turned an alarming cash outlay into a positive. Had I called it a plaything or a mere vehicle on which I could parade my incredible physique (ahem), it may have been considered extravagant - at least by my wife, who needs some new slippers. No, this was part of my 'keep-out-of-a-hole-in-the-ground' master plan, alternatively named 'Operation Pork', so worth every penny. If I do happen to snuff it Jan can sell the bike and get a few flowers.

On a similar theme Jan and I had a conversation the other day discussing new teeth. Mine look like a building site and hers, though much better, are showing signs of wear. I said, 'New screw-in teeth would cost about twenty thousand for a set, which is a hell of an outlay.'

'If you die I could always sell them,' she replied. 'I could put them on Gum Tree.'

The timing of my new regime is particularly convenient because I'm currently on an alcoholiday – a month off the wine. I need to look after myself and take things cautiously because I have ten litres of indeterminate boxed red in stock and have no intention of croaking it and leaving a wine lake to someone who won't appreciate it!

6

A Slope and a Hedge

The battery is fully charged - that took 4 hours. I've repaired my puncture - that took half an hour and cost £17! I'll explain that cock-up in due course but now it's time to introduce Columbanus to his new world. It is a 'he' by the way, largely because, like men in general, he doesn't listen. To get any response I need to feed him precise instructions, slowly.

It's barely light as I leave the launch pad. The hour is carefully planned to frustrate prying eyes (turns out it's a good job). I'm trying to avoid headlines like: *'Local hero looks like a complete pillock.'* Sir Chris Hoy I am not – witness ...

I make an utter hash of coming off the drive. I'm wearing a nasty, light-green reflective top, the kind of thing all the trendiest pedallers wear, but I'm a bit sketchy in the trouser department. They are old jogging bottoms. They've never been jogged in, but they have done plenty of gardening. Past their best is generous. They are saggy.

The power control consists of 'Off, 1, 2, 3' depicted by little LED lights. I've set it on number 1. Easing into things, you realize. It all works thus: when you press down on the pedal the *'motor assist'* kicks in after a slight delay, half a second perhaps. In mode 1 there's not a massive power boost, but it's certainly noticeable. From the front of our house to the avenue it's downhill quite steeply for about 15 yards, so any acceleration is enhanced by the slope.

So ... picture this if you will. The left pedal is raised. I stand on it with my left foot, and my weight naturally pushes down the pedal. As the bike starts to move, the motor kicks in. I go to hoist my right leg over the seat in order to locate my foot on the right pedal. Simple. Just like riding a bike.

Unfortunately, my saggy jogging bottoms get stuck on the back of the saddle so I can't get my leg over. I'm now sprawled along the bike, accelerating down the slope, enhanced by the motor, utterly out of control. I'm lying along the length of the bike, rather like a head-first skeleton rider on the Cresta Run. I hurtle, speed increasing exponentially, straight across the avenue into my neighbour's hedge.

It's six in the morning and I wonder whether I'm doing the right thing.

These are the hard yards. You'll have seen Olympic rowers winning gold in the summer sun, but the real hard graft is done on sleety winter mornings in the pre-dawn murk on the wave-beaten waters of the Thames. Endless hours honing technique and physique. Well, if being tangled up in my neighbour's privet hedge is the price I have to pay for gliding god-like around the neighbourhood, then so be it.

I leave Columbanus propped up against the hedge and go and change into something less saggy before I kill myself. A lesson learned. Luckily, we live on a quiet avenue where there is still 3 hours before people get moving. I've not been spotted. I reflect that it's a good job we don't live near a railway line or motorway from where hordes of gawping commuters could get their working day off to a chuckling start. But, if nothing else, I have learned to treat my new bike with respect. It's a machine, after all, and if my instructions are inaccurate I can expect difficulties.

So, suitably attired, off we go. I've planned to do a six-miler - the same route I regularly walk. The handbook tells me the battery will be good for up to 45km depending on the amount of 'assistance' I use. I suspect this will probably be quite a lot, at least to begin with. I've half a mile of main roads to cover before I get to the canal towpath. The bike has an integral headlight and a small flashing red rear light, which I had to buy extra. In addition to my unpleasant reflective top, I also have reflective bits on pedals and helmet. But I still feel like a sacrificial target for motorists, even the few that are about at around six in the morning. I'm used to travelling in a car and had largely forgotten how being exposed like this is unsettling. In fact, I think all motorists should experience the raw noise and power of their vehicles close up to appreciate just how much potential danger they are wielding in their silenced cocoons. Just drive with the window down for a while and you'll soon understand, particularly if there are trucks and buses about.

Stop raving, you idiot - you're supposed to be enjoying your new-found freedom.

I go a couple of miles along the canal, including going up alongside 7 or 8 locks. These are steep little bits that previously caused me to really struggle. Now, on power setting two, I fly up them. Frankly, it's marvellous. This is a zooming day where the capabilities of my steed are being tested. Other days will be pottering days when I will take in my surroundings and actually enjoy it. And I'll be able to see it - it's still dark right now! In the days before battery power I needed to concentrate on just getting home, so some of the finer points of the local sights passed me by, albeit pretty slowly!

There is a ¾-mile lockless section at the summit of the Rochdale Canal which I zip along at 15 miles per hour, except when I pass dog walkers or walkers without dogs, not that there are many at six in the morning. Being a walker myself, I know that a bike can be threatening on a narrow towpath, so I slow right down when we pass. I go slowly enough so they can see I'm an old fart and little threat. Some even bid me good morning and say thank you.

The next stage is up over a disused section of B-road. Fairly steep, but again I shoot up it. It's a pity the crowds are not lining the roadside to cheer me on with their motorhomes, flags and a thousand bikes. It's a short-cut I used to take to work many years ago. Thankfully it's now impassable for cars because the council has failed to maintain the road and it's crumbling down the hillside. Nowadays its a rare safe haven for cyclists and walkers. Nature is taking over. It's peculiar seeing road-signs, once of real importance, now semi-obscured by foliage. In fact, it's a treat to see nature reclaiming a space rather than us destroying it and building houses. It's a pity this stretch is only a little over half a mile long.

Over the summit and down the other side I rejoin 'public' highway again and realize what an appalling state our road surfaces are in. Parts of it are seriously dangerous for bikes. Mine has fat off-road tyres but I could envisage thin road-bike tyres having a real problem. Of course, you can steer round a pothole, but you can't when there's a bus up your rear end and vehicles coming the other way! Apart from a scuff on my wrist from my visit to the hedge the only other injury this trip is when I stop quickly and dismount so a bus can come through a narrow gap towards me. I scrape my shin painfully on a pedal so I'm using some pretty outdoor language as I hobble home. But, back home we are and trip number one is under the belt. Verdict: great! I plug in the charger and no tyres deflate. Things are looking up.

Note to self: better get a first aid kit.

7

Upwardly Mobile (slowly...)

Remember the £17 puncture repair? I order some kit (patches and tyre levers) and present myself at Halfords, purveyor of motor car spares and cycling equipment. Except I forget my phone which has confirmation of my order, so the bloke has to enter everything into the computer manually again. Technology is all well and good - it's supposed to make things easier - but there's danger in letting an old git loose with anything more complicated than a piece of string. Problems may ensue. In this instance the man in the shop ends up muttering to himself while I feel a bit inadequate. It's not like he's busy, though; there's nobody else in the bike section, which is the whole first floor of the modern retail unit.

There's almost no stock either. It looks like someone has ransacked the place, rather like a moonscape. I wander around trying to look like a cyclist. Had I not recently bought a bike I wouldn't have got one here either. My choice is limited to a small lady's bike which is non-electric and pink, or a selection of junior bikelets with stabilizers.

£7 for the repair kit and tyre levers. 'You don't need glue - the patches are self-adhesive,' he replies to my enquiry. Frankly I feel a bit of a knob even asking for glue. Things have moved on since I last repaired a puncture. Idiot-proof self-adhesive patches nowadays. Remember years ago when we did use glue? It spurted out the side of the patch and stuck your fingers to the tyre, then crusted on your finger ends. Did we use talcum powder or some such to stop the glued patch sticking to the tyre itself? Or chalk? Can't remember, but there's none of that nonsense in today's world of speed and convenience.

As I'm leaving, the assistant shouts across the warehouse, 'You could have bought 4 new inner tubes for a tenner, you know. It's a limited offer.' Now he tells me! Anyhow, was it an impulse buy? Maybe, but I bought four! The cheapness of inner tubes is why Paul's assistant suggested I buy one rather than a repair kit. I apologise retrospectively for calling him. Perhaps if he'd explained ...? Back in my garage I effect my repair. Repair note, not replacement: I'd bought the kit and was damn well going to use it! Glueless patches and all.

In the corner, malevolently watching me repair its replacement, is my stepdaughter's mountain bike. I feel sorry for it; the poor thing deserves better. In my hands it is the personification of potential unfulfilled. A 'Mountain' bike it certainly wasn't. I scuttled along flat areas like a corpulent beetle. If it's possible to waddle on a bicycle, I did it. I shall return it to its more deserving owner as soon as possible.

* * *

OK, Columbanus, time to show what you can do. Let's go up on the moors. The A58 is a trans-Pennine route that connects Lancashire and Yorkshire. The crest of the hill is known as Blackstone Edge. I can actually see the pub that marks the summit from my bedroom window. It's like waking up in a hotel in Zermatt and seeing wispy clouds whipping across the summit of the Matterhorn (nearly). My climb is slightly less arduous but it is about two and a half miles long and rises around eight hundred feet. I think it's deemed to be a category 3 climb. Now that sounds pretty impressive, despite the fact that I've no idea what it means. What I do know is that it's pretty incessant from the outset, a climb that I would have no chance of doing without battery assistance. Well, I could do it, but with lots of breaks and it would be (metaphorically) dark by the time I got to the top. At around 150 feet I pass The Moorcock Inn, a hostelry I visit from time to time. As I wheeze past, I can't deny there's a temptation ...

Being Lancastrian (and more obviously humanoid than 'folk from York-shire') I consider the A58 to be an umbilical cord through which we can nourish our less fortunate neighbours. Conveniently there is a non-return valve to prevent a load of old pudding coming the other way. We don't want to compromise our gene pool after all. As chance would have it, the actual county border is a little way past the summit. If you're smart you can get to the top, enjoy the benefits of lovely views and fresh air (that has been known to come in the form of a gale), have a nice meal at The White House pub and still avoid Yorkshire altogether!

So, I leave civilization behind and up we go. Even though the bike is electric I still have to pedal. If you stop pedalling, the motor cuts out. Shortly after that, due to the effects of gravity, the bike would come to a stop and I would fall over sideways. Don't assume that there's no effort involved; there is, and by the time I've reached the pub at the top my thighs are really burning - and that's with the bike in its lowest gear most of the time and on full assist. It's taken about twenty-five minutes. That is pathetic to anybody who is young, fit and has decent equipment (legs) but for me it's an achievement, so please don't take the piss. I fared marginally better than the badger that's decomposing on the verge halfway up.

A couple of hours later, when the dizziness has moderated, I have the choice of zooming down the hill again or doing some pottering. Surprisingly perhaps, there's plenty of battery left, so a potter it is. Just past the pub I can turn left in front of Blackstone Edge Reservoir and travel the gravel service roads that connect several hill-top reservoirs. The views are spectacular, not least because when you're on the crest of a hill the valley below is hidden. It's like standing on top of the Duomo in Florence where things immediately below are hidden by the curve of the roof. In other words, we can look across to distant hillsides as if nothing man-made exists. I can imagine our forebears travelling these moors in magnificent isolation. Straw-coloured tussocky grass shimmers in the wind, a natural blanket warming centuries-old peat. You have to mentally block out the electricity pylons, though. Boy, does man make such a mess of things. There's more 'Pylon News' later! If I look into the valley far below I can see the last remaining patches of green. I'm trying to make the most of it because they will soon be buried under concrete.

8

Now and Then

In the newsagent a while ago, a headline on the front of a women's magazine caught my eye: *'Do you comfort eat? It could be down to your cycle.'* That was enough, I didn't read any more and sold my bike. You can't be too careful, I thought – temptation, get rid!

I was a bit rash, really - I missed the bike. A year or two later I was still comfort eating but still not exercising! There was little mirth at the size of my girth, so that's partly why I'm having another go on two wheels. Yes, I'm happy to be enjoying biking again, lucky to have a second chance doing something I used to enjoy so much. Thanks to Columbanus, I am once again a spring chicken on wheels (or cock of the north). Pre the electric era I used to cycle quite a lot - often ten miles per day, sometimes thirty or so. Usually early in the morning at first light, any time from 4.00 AM. Silent, me time. Not quite silent - there was quite a lot of me huffing and puffing between the hedgerows.

In the depths of rural France, I'd just set off on tiny country roads and see where they led. I operated in kilometers on the continent because it sounded further and on downhill stretches I could get into double figures kph. I'd come across small villages or farms, silent and apparently lifeless, save for a snoozing dog; sometimes a large ivy-clad country house with window shutters to fend off summer heat; occasionally a chateau with moat and stables surrounded by woodland and accessed by a pale, tree-lined drive;

magical rides when I'd never know what was next. I was confident that, no matter how far I went or how lost I got, I'd get back.

One time, in a place called Genelard, a small commune in Burgundy, I discovered a four-kilometer circuit which I used to circumnavigate three times. Travelling at what I thought a respectable pace, I was passed one time by a group of six leather-skinned old men - one group of many fit, reptilian creatures that stalk the rural French byways. They must have been eighty if they were a day! All were lean, helmeted and Lycra-clad; a gay kaleidoscope of yellows, blues and reds. Some sported orthopaedic braces on knees or elbows. I was given a series of 'bonjours' as they whipped past in a cloud of ancient after-shave and liniment. Had I been competitive I could have put on a spurt and re-passed them, leaving them in a noxious cloud of fags and red wine. It would have been a heck of an effort, though, which would have seen me spent for the day – or longer. In the end I decided to remain at comfortable cruising speed.

We all take things for granted, but we shouldn't. We could do with an early warning system that reminds us to enjoy the moment. Don't take 'now' for granted because 'now' is all we have to look back on. We need to look back and say 'Wow, 'now' was good.' Then we can get on with making some more memories for tomorrow. I'm creating memories through walking and biking. And I'm actually looking where I'm going, seeing my home town and surroundings (of some 60 years) properly for the first time. It's all too easy to scoot past things without looking and wondering. For example, one of the reservoirs I walk and ride round is called Hollingworth Lake. Until I took note I had no idea that Captain Webb practiced here. Remember him? He was the first person to swim the English Channel back in 1875. The Channel is some 300 miles distant from our Lake. It's also bloody cold, like the Channel. Funnily enough, Captain Webb was born in Dawley, Shropshire. We lived near there for a while! Strange world, eh? The more you delve the stranger things get.

There's no right or wrong way to experience things, but at this point in my journey I'm dawdling. More accurately, it's a mixture of cantering and dawdling. In other words, when something of potential interest comes up I 'come down off the canter' and dawdle. Sometimes it's a bit of an effort to get back up to the canter again.

Early morning there is a mixture of Lycra-clad beauties and old gits, like me. I consider myself to be at the second awkward age. The first is adolescence when gangly limbs and spots are the problem; this latter one causes more fundamental difficulties, such as whether I can get my leg over the crossbar without lying the bike on its side; or gazing out over the magnificent sun-dappled moors wondering whether I've taken my 75mg Aspirin.

People jog to get fit. Most seem wrapped in an electronic world, focused solely on the next step (solely ... foot ... jogging – well, I never ...!). Everything else is bypassed - journey's end is their kitchen, happy to be quad-stretching and sweaty after their exertion while the world beyond rolls on. Unnoticed by our jogger the birds sing, the foxes screech and Captain Webb trains.

Mind you, not even an e-bike can get the better of a British winter. Yesterday it was barely above freezing and slippery under foot; today it's 4 degrees and there's horizontal sleet whipping across at 30 mph - conditions truly the enemy of the cyclist. These are the days I walk instead. I can skip from bus shelter to tree to doorway like Inspector Clouseau sneaking after his suspect through Parisian Streets. Not now, Cato!!

9

The Best Laid Plans ... of Nice Old Men

Last week, sixty years ago, I celebrated my first birthday. Well, not personally ... I just sort of lay there whinging. Rather unfairly, everyone else got pickled. From the safety of my pram, I vowed never to be left out again. But, way back when, I was the pride of my parents, a blank canvas.

My 1st and 61st birthdays have something in common. I can remember very little about them, despite the recent one being only a week ago! One thing I do remember is that Jan gave me a pair of binoculars - a great present for a cyclist with 61-year-old eyes. They will open up distant vistas and allow me to see things far away at any given moment; birds or deer that previously have been moving smudges in the distance will spring to life in abundant glory (maybe). Thankfully, my binoculars won't let me see into the future - I don't want to know what's coming, thank you very much. Chances are I wouldn't be able to change much even if I wanted to. It's now I need to focus on. Of course, that doesn't mean we can't prepare some short / medium-term blueprints ...

Travel and the planning of trips has been difficult for the past pandemic year. The coming months will be far from certain, too. So, because longer jaunts, including staying away for a day or two, may not be possible I thought we'd focus on shorter day trips - zippy little fun-filled forays where we can all join in. Jan tells me she fancies visiting country houses - National Trust properties, for example. We won't be able to go inside but we can mooch round the grounds. Sounds good - we can combine that with me having a cycle, both of us having a good dog walk and, if the weather allows, a picnic. See?! Sounds like a plan. Things are looking up.

Step one requires a vehicle upgrade. The previous one has been used as a builder's wagon for five house renovations and is looking rather the worse for wear. In fact, we have to wipe our feet before we get out. It's got one or two alarming rattles and the key fob only works if I bash it on the roof rack a few times (which itself is rusted on). I reckon we'll need something quite large to accommodate me, Jan, the dog (in a cage), Columbanus (my bike), assorted paraphernalia and a picnic.

Turns out my bike is huge compared to regular mountain bikes; short of buying a mid-size van, I'd have to remove various bits to get it in - whatever car we buy. I don't want it on a rack externally for fear of getting it pinched. Anyhow, we traded in my SUV (Squalid Unkempt Vauxhall) for a 7-seat MPV (Mean Platelet Volume - thank you, Google). I've folded away the third row of seats permanently, folded down the second row temporarily and we now have a warehouse on wheels.

I've had mixed success with cars and things over the years. It started when I failed the theory part of my driving test (it was just a few questions back then at the end of the driving bit). The examiner asked me what signposts I might expect on a country road. 'Pick your own strawberries' apparently wasn't the answer he was looking for, so I was advised to go and brush up on the technical side.

Our old car had never let us down, despite the punishment I gave it. It's now worth £150, which is approximately 10 times less than my new bike, but I was offered £350 as a trade-in and they knocked a grand off the new one - so the deal was sealed. If the new (to us) car is as reliable as the Astra, I'll be more than happy.

* * *

Time for a trial trip. We chose Clitheroe in Lancashire. Bit random in a way, but

I'd discovered a house for sale, one we could look at, and it's in our permitted Covid travel area. My train of thought has been affected by lockdown because we didn't actually want to move house. The excitement of leaving the avenue got both of us in a tizz. It was like we were off to the Great Barrier Reef. Instead, to make our trip rather more jazzy, we decided we were going to the Cake District (Chorley is not far away).

Anyway, I remove my bike's front wheel and seat and in it goes. (Boy, it's not half heavy and there's a nasty twinge around my L4 vertebrae as I heave it in.) Dog cage, dog, extraneous bits plus picnic all follow into the back. Me and Jan in the front. Full of hope, we set off. We arrive in Clitheroe to discover the house is dreadful and the dog has been sick on the picnic hamper. Not in any violent 'tiger roaring out of the undergrowth way' - no, surreptitiously. But enough to be slightly off-putting. He was anxious about being in a smart new car, I think. He is more used to gamboling around in plasterboard dust.

Refusing to be downhearted, we decide to go to Lytham St. Annes because I want to look at the sea and my aunt and uncle used to live there. Spurious reasoning again, I think. I can't tell you how cold it is. There's a biting wind howling in off the Irish Sea, so I won't be getting the bike out here! We promenade on the sea front with a veritable tide of fellow geriatrics, muffled-up citizens waddling north and south by the sea-abandoned sands. We have a brew and a lump of cheese from a mini-market and return home to clean the car!

To be honest, I'm not keen on things getting off to too good a start. Inevitably, they have to go downhill and you can get blasé. I'm a great believer that if things start badly it's a positive. To a degree, of course; if you ride over a cliff on your first outing, that's not good. My first brief ride ended up in a privet hedge so I took that to be a good omen, long-term. I look forward to our next trip out in the warehouse.

10

Dutch Ditch

I t's 2007, late September, and I'm in the Netherlands. I love this country, but I'm feeling rather too English. I feel the need to integrate more. The natives use specially developed vocal chords to speak a language that has too many consonants. The resulting sound is a guttural, throat-clearing rasp. The language and its deployment is quite beyond me. Thankfully, many Dutch people speak English so I'm not completely isolated. But it's friendship on their say-so.

They are a tall race, whereas I am not; nor is Jan. In fact, anyone over the age of 4 is taller than me. To illustrate this point, we were in a hotel up in Friesland when Jan got stuck in a monstrous bath. It must have been half as big again as a regular one and, being soapy, she just couldn't get any purchase to lever herself out. She was marooned. Even the loo was a few inches higher than normal. All very uncomfortable. I think they probably put us in the room specially designed for giants out of spite because Jan had negotiated a substantial discount on the room. Our cuisines are different though both, in part, good. I like their meatballs, and snert (a hazardous pea and ham soup that kills you. Er, sorry ... I mean, is to die for).

At this early stage of our continental odyssey, we don't appear to have much in common with the natives. One thing we do share, on a national basis, is appalling weather. Having said that, our temporary home town is called Zwartsluis , which is located in the centre, north of the Netherlands. It is some way south of our home town near Manchester, but despite this it seems to get consistently colder. Regularly minus double figures, which is not much good for a weed like me. But there is one area where I can join in ... cycling. It is a BIG pastime and an important part of the Dutch way of life.

From the outset I decide I wanted to look like a proper cyclist in the land of proper cyclists. I no longer wish to be the lethargic relation, wheezing and rattling along in the slipstream of the gods. In short, I don't want to look English. Somehow, we don't appear to make much of a sartorial effort, so we have tended to stand out a bit. Still do! We have this demeanour that looks alien on foreign soil. Some of us are worse than others; holiday-makers can be the most stand-out - the budget flight lands in Ibiza and here they come: white legs, black socks and plastic sandals lurching across the apron towards the nearest bar ... you get the picture.

Me? Well, despite making some effort, most of the time I look like a particularly disadvantaged refugee. Somehow I always look a bit 'knotted hanky.' It's my shape, you see. The gents' outfitters of today just don't make clothes for the perfect figure. Things rarely hang right.

* * *

I bought my bike second-hand. Not just second-hand, probably many more. The local bike emporium has an end-of-season sale each autumn. There is a huge variety of bikes, both in specification and price. Some are ex-demonstrators, high-tech electric machines which are ahead of their time really - at least ten years ahead of the 'E' popularity surge in the UK.

Top-notch bicycles are reduced from a retail price of around €1200 to perhaps €500. That's a heck of a saving, and the bikes are damn near perfect. The problem is we're coming into the northerly Dutch winter when it gets very chilly, as I've said - not really cycling weather. Of course, there are better (less cold) days, but you still won't get full value for your bike. Being flat, there is usually a wind blowing. From any angle you're liable to be buffeted by gusts of varying ferocity and temperature. The one you really need to avoid is the northerly or nor'easter, beasts that gather chill and intensity somewhere around the Baltic and whip in over the flat landscape with savage force. Those can be very unpleasant.

This was the era before my leg problems, so I didn't even consider an electric bike. The one I got wasn't reduced in price. In fact, it was increased - from around zero to €40 when they put some air in the tyres. Just for show the proprietor thought he'd better charge me something. I'd found it languishing close to the back fence behind some sorry-looking children's tricycles - but I recognized its potential. It appears that the Dutch prefer things new to used, and that includes bikes, so there's lots of second-hand ones around for us thrifty Englanders.

Now this, let me tell you, was a pretty good machine. It had more gears than I would ever need and the paintwork was fine; in fact, everything worked perfectly - even the bell, which was a polite continental 'boing' as opposed to an annoying towpath 'ting.' It's just that had it been standing next to its more glamorous cousins it would have, well, dragged the display down a bit. Looked rather English, if you will. The shopkeeper made sure my purchase was completed in all haste lest he be seen handling a machine that was 'dragging the average down.' The thing is that when I'm flashing around at high speed nobody will be able to tell what my bike really looks like; I'll simply be going too fast! Or I could disguise myself by wearing an Arab thawb - then I'd be a wolf in Sheikh's clothing.

I return to the shop (without my bike to spare his blushes) to buy a few extras - drinks holder, water bottle and the like. I don't need to do much to Europhy my cycling look (new word there - make me look European, in other words). I decide one thing that would make me look (in)credible is triathlon bars. Know what I mean? The forward-facing looped frame attached to the handlebars, allowing you to lean forward on your forearms, hands out in front. An altogether a more streamlined look - more elite athlete, less ... well ... Lancastrian.

* * *

The Netherlands is geared up for cycling. Geared up, huh! Alongside the highways are purpose-built cycle lanes, often one each side of the road. Even if they're just on one side, there's plenty of room for two bikes to pass, providing the other rider is slimmer than me. You're safely out of the traffic, and being perched up on a bike you can see for miles. It's pleasant cycling on tracks that are, in the main, beautifully maintained. There are even proper white line markings at roundabouts where cycles have priority over cars. In other words, if a car wants to turn right off a roundabout it has to give way to cyclists who are going straight on. Woe betide the car driver who knocks a cyclist off. The cycle is King.

Road maintenance is good; any problems seem to be rectified quickly. So, picture the scene as I trundle through the countryside ... Half the road is closed for repairs so there are temporary traffic lights. The roadworks affect the cycle lane too, so they have built a mini-diversion for cyclists. The temporary cycle path turns sharp right, left, left, then right again. Three sides of a rectangle round the work site.

I'm hurtling along, sprawled along my triathlon bars, head down, in a state of cycling euphoria. I feel very fortunate - it's only the supreme athlete (*ahem*) who gets to experience this harmonic rhapsody of man and machine. I look up just in time to be faced with a red plastic barrier. Here I need to register a mini-complaint. A design shortfall of triathlon bars is that they don't have brake levers. It wouldn't have mattered in this case anyway, because I'd looked up too late, far too late to adjust my grip and reach the brakes on the handlebars proper. I arrived at pace at the barrier, which was more robust than it looked. In fact, it stayed still while I kept going.

The line of cars waiting at the temporary lights saw me collide with the bright red obstruction and sail over the handlebars. I wasn't airborne for long but did have time to glimpse a wide-eyed native watching me from the comfort of his stationary Audi. He saw a pudgy, Lycra-clad missile disappear from view straight into a big hole, followed almost immediately by his flying machine.

I was lucky that the hole was muddy rather than rocky, so my landing was relatively gentle. Audi man helped me out. Once he realized I wasn't dead he smiled a bit - as Dutch people do when they get to know you. Very sportingly, he gave me a lift home - my clothing ripped, a bit bloody, my bike bent. Perhaps he was a cyclist himself, recognizing a fellow icon of the road in a pickle.

Looks like I might have to part with €40 for another bike. I wonder if they do trade-ins. Actually, after a rub down with *The Dutch Cycling Times* and a new front wheel (pinched from another wreck in the compound) my bike was back to its original state. (I nearly said back to it's best then, but that would probably have been twenty years ago). I was away again, full of enthusiasm but watchful for holes.

11

Bike with Brains

Columbanus is an amazing machine; he seems to know when I need help. He can sense distress. Not sure how it works in all honesty, but he seems to increase his power input the more I need it; the steeper the hill, the more the boost. Maybe he can hear me wheezing or sense my nausea. On the flat he all but turns himself off. Downhill, he knows I don't need help so he goes into huff mode and won't work.

Motor assistance is limited to 15 mph. If you get to 15 on a bike it's fun and exhilarating, but mine is not really designed for speed; it's a mountain bike after all, designed for rugged terrain. Picture those photos from a glossy cycling mag where a supreme physical specimen leaps over a jump, handlebars and frame misaligned like steering into an airborne skid. The backdrop? A tree-clad range of mountains defined by chalk-white, precipitous cliffs. Yes, quite right, that's not me …

My 'big hill' route is three miles up. I tackle that at conservative speed in first or second gears (mostly first, actually). Coming down I reach 35 miles an hour. Not that quick, particularly for a road bike (or racing bike as we used to call them) but quite fast enough for a chunky-tyred mountain bike. If any of you have driven a caravan, perhaps you've experienced that unpleasant wobbly motion where the van becomes unstable and starts to veer from side to side. I'm a bit like that. My rear end becomes unstable at (relatively) high speed, particularly if I'm cornering. I do get a bit of a thrill out of a descent, usually just after it's over and I've survived.

The wind howls through my jowls and my eyes water. My flobby bits joggle about like a hyperthermic jelly and I lose sensation in my frozen feet. I did toy with the idea of wrap-around glasses, likely blue, but realized I probably looked enough of a dickhead already. Due to my watering eyes I have an idea what Eddie 'The Eagle' Edwards felt like hurtling down his ski jump with impaired visibility.

I met Eddie many years ago. What a decent, thoroughly nice guy he is. And courage? Well, he had a shot at life and took it. He was portrayed as a glorious failure, but not in my eyes. He had more bottle than anyone I have ever met. His Olympics was 1988. (And it was his - can you remember anyone else who competed?) I visited Calgary a couple of years after him and saw in the distance the ski jumps he tackled, both 70- and 90-metre hills. It was summertime and they looked unnaturally skeletal and misplaced. I have actually viewed a 90-metre hill from the top (in Norway). It looks miles down to the run-off area where the crowd gathers. The actual landing area is just about as steep as the jump itself. And looking down, I can tell you it is mighty steep and a heck of a long way to the bottom. Anyone who sets off on that particular journey has oodles of courage or a screw loose. Or both. Looking at the Calgary jumps from distance, I got goose bumps and had a sense of real pride that one of ours had lit up the Winter Olympics.

If Eddie had come down my hill on my bike, I get the feeling he would have gone a bit faster, loved it a bit more and smiled more broadly. I'm slightly cowardly to be fair. Not sure how well the body would heal these days in the event of an accident, so I'm slightly circumspect. But I still get a thrill.

The off-road capability does come in handy around my home town of Littleborough because the roads surfaces are so appalling. The other day, one youngster playing hopscotch on a side street hopped straight down a pothole and disappeared from sight. They needed the fire brigade to get her out.

When I'm weary my bike senses it and rubs salt into the wounds. He somehow makes me crave a slice or two of honey-roast ham and a glass of Merlot – and at that point, as if by reciprocal telekinesis, we turn for home and the succour of the larder. But Columbanus has lazy days when he's not up for it and sometimes I have to put my foot down (then the other). Occasionally I have to bully him to leave the avenue where we live. He claims charging issues or low tyre pressure. It would be too easy to fall for his deception but I have to be strong. Determined. You don't earn the label 'elite' pottering around your own avenue.

Yes, I say 'we' because we're a team. Columbanus would be pretty useless without me and I would be considerably slower and more knackered without him. And speaking of knackered, here is a description unkindly attested of me by my brother. He is able to ignore the mass of superlative adjectives available to capture my athleticism and simply describes me as 'a knackered bloke on a bike ...' Not wholly inaccurate if the truth be known, though there are other combinations of those words that may equally suit. For example ...

If I've driven into a wall ...

Bloke on a knackered bike ...

If I've overdone it ...

Bloke, knackered, on a bike ...

If I fall off ...

Bike on a knackered bloke ...

If I fall off at high speed (which is unlikely) ...

Bike, knackered, on a bloke.

It's not easy this cycling business, so I leave the technical aspects of our sorties to Columbanus, the brains of the outfit.

12

Bicycles and Icicles

The permafrost is slowly releasing its grip. The ice-sheet drifts slowly north, crackling its way towards Scotland. Here in Lancashire, we are left with the soggy remnants of winter. Last year's unpruned plants sit grey and bedraggled, like one of my culinary creations dumped in the garden by a discerning dinner guest.

Winter can be the enemy of the cyclist, particularly one with dodgy feet. Despite multi-layers of socks, the cold still penetrates. I've tried socks from the world over in an attempt to keep warm. The best I found were from Germany, but since Brexit they are 'unavailable.' My tootsies are a victim of Britain's go-it-alone revolution. But, a silver lining! I've found a replacement supplier who offers British-made, multi-coloured, knee-length 'ski' socks. If nothing else, they look very smart. I haven't tried them out in anger yet because it's chucking it down and my e-bike is unsuited to wet conditions.

This raises two questions. Should not a bicycle be sufficiently water-resistant to be ridden in the rain? Do I want to ride in the rain? The answer to the second one is no, so question one is irrelevant.

Actually, I did buy a pair of cycling overshoes, Velcro-fastened, that you slip over your shoes. They supposedly keep out the damp and the cold. By the time I'd insulated myself with multi-layers of weatherproof clothing it was a real struggle to even bend down. And as I finally made it, the sheer physical effort precipitated an enormous cramp in my Taylor's muscle. Also called the Sartorius muscle, it's a big thing that runs down the inner thigh and is very painful when cramped. Before I'd even got going I was hobbling around the garage cursing sub-standard equipment (legs). Most people get cramps following exercise. I think it just demonstrates my extraordinary level of fitness that the slightest movement can have such calamitous effects.

In winter I often return from my early morning trundle to sit with my feet on a microwaved bean bag while eating my breakfast sardines. My friend and neighbour turns his nose up at my choice of morning fuel. But what's the difference between fish at lunch or fish in the morning? Yes, it's 'early doors' when I digest my shortcomings and evaluate my (lack of) progress. As my poor old body realigns itself, and to stretch the fishy metaphor, I trawl over that morning's achievements (or lack of) and ponder how I could do it better. Buy a motorcycle, perhaps? Or a car?

First thing in the morning you can get away with things. Remember my encounter with my neighbour's hedge? Accomplished (I use that word advisedly) under cover of darkness while my senior neighbours slumbered on. Had the same incident occurred in sight of a busload of locals I may have given up cycling there and then. The loss of face may have been too much to bear.

I also see some peculiar things first thing. I encountered an acquaintance one morning, a man I usually see during the afternoon. He's not an early morning person at all. When I bumped into him he grumbled that his alarm had gone off 'unexpectedly' and he was unable to get back to sleep. Deciding to take the dog out was evidently a mistake for both him and the reluctant hound. I discovered somebody camping on the bowling green one day. A tent, with attendant paraphernalia, stood in magnificent isolation right in the middle of the green. I posted a photo on the local website but nobody responded. A fabrication, people would have thought. But no, somebody had seen a patch of neatly mown grass and 'gone for it.'

The weather here in the Pennine foothills can be unpredictable. That's being polite. I often set off in the dark and can see the stars. This indicates that precipitation is unlikely. At least imminently. But squally showers can sneak up and in the blink of an eye you suddenly find yourself riding into gusty sleet. Or is that sleety gusts? Whichever, neither is very pleasant. And it's the feet that take the brunt. But I've tried out my new ski socks and they have passed the test. They are part-wool with a bit of stretchy stuff in them. As you'd expect from ski socks they are better at going downhill; in that respect we are well-matched.

Other extremities suffer, but not to the same degree. My face is usually red and blotchy but it's unclear whether it's the weather or the wine. I need to do more research. My fingers get chilled but I wear two pairs of gloves – a pair of cycling ones underneath a double-layered thermo pair. I used to have some silky inners, too, but the mice in the garage ate them.

Incidentally, the cycling gloves have special fingertip pads that allow me to operate my touch-screen phone without taking them off. I've not used this feature yet. In fact, the only occasion I can envisage using it is following brake failure on my 3-mile descent when I may need to call an ambulance in anticipation of the inevitable crash.

Early morning winter cycling can be a bit of a gamble. Columbanus is equipped with a pretty good front light, which frankly is essential to avoid potholes. I sometimes take a slightly unnerving route that includes a tree-lined stretch of the Rochdale Canal. Wet leaves on a bitumen towpath, which is narrow, can be the cyclist's enemy. My light illuminates a bright patch right in front but I'm aware that a couple of feet to my left is the cold (sometimes frozen) canal. It's just a dark void and not a place I want to go. Every now and then the water reflects a wink of light from my headlight or the moon, reminding me that danger lurks. An added problem is that the carpet of leaves can hide stones or bits of rubble, or ruts or potholes. The darkest stretch is just over a mile, so caution is exercised.

Last time I went this route I nearly met a sticky end for another reason. After the canal stretch I turn left up a hill. The road is quite narrow but busy with early-morning commuters. As I climb, a van is passing me and there's another coming the other way. There's not much spare room and I'm concentrating hard when a dog being walked along the footpath takes exception to me, lunges on its lead and nips my trouser leg. Very alarming, and I'm not sure how I didn't swerve into the path of the van. I called the dog-owner an unpleasant name that rhymed with bat. But, as is the convention these days, rather than apologising she went on the attack and blamed me for startling her rat. (I didn't call her a rat).

Spurred on by the promise of sardines, I stow my lack of dignity in my children's rucksack and speed off up the hill like a wobbly green blob. My battery-assisted buttocks leave the woman and her murderous dog in the dust. Yes, children's rucksack. It looked bigger in the advert, but it's big enough for my binoculars, plus spare inner tube and an emergency lump of cheddar.

13

Bank in Birmingham

I n Birmingham, England's second city, I *almost* had a very nasty coming-together with a large local man. I say local ... I just presumed because he looked to meld into the place; huge, solid - like the city itself. If he'd told me he was a local I would have accepted it; to have done otherwise would have courted confrontation, and he would win! As it was, he never actually spoke. However, despite him not uttering one word, there was a physical coming-together of sorts. Thank goodness it didn't develop into fisticuffs or I may well have needed emergency medical intervention. Allow me to expand ...

I normally ride around cities in the early morning, but occasionally I'm forced into a daytime foray and, as a result, do battle with Mr and Mrs Normal, who live during normal hours in a normal house, as sensible people do. Anyhow, just after three in the afternoon we arrived, on our boat, at the Gas Street Basin canal moorings. We needed cash urgently so I had to dash to the bank. By the time I'd lumped the bike off the roof and got organised, it was uncomfortably near closing time. Plus, I wasn't quite sure where I was going. I was aiming for an address near the Bullring and had to ask directions of a number of people, only some of whom spoke the same language as me. Of those that did, some were clueless visitors and others seemed reluctant to help a yellow sphere in a blue cycling helmet.

I arrived about five minutes before closing time. Bank closing time, that is -

the time when most people are at work and unable to avail themselves of the bank's services. The banks need a couple of hours to cash up, I suppose. And time to have meetings to make sure the interest rates on offer the following day erode our savings at a satisfactory rate.

At the foot of a couple of steps in front of the bank there's a row of bikes parked in a long cycle rack. I hurriedly secure my bike with plastic-enclosed chain and padlock and dash in to join the back of a long, slow-moving queue. I've moved on a pace or two when the doors close behind me and entry to further customers is halted. An employee is engaged to release those who have completed their business but keep new arrivals out - thus separated from their own money.

When I emerge after about twenty minutes, I see a very large man, with the physique of a prize-winning wrestler, standing staring at my bike with his hands on his hips. Huge shoulders, small waist, jeans, tight t-shirt. Every few moments he raises his head and looks around him. I think to myself, surely this bugger's not thinking about stealing my bike?! I approach with caution and say 'hi' from a safe distance. He turns and looks at me, then back down at the bike. Keeping his head still, saying nothing, his eyes flick between me and the bike. Then I see why. I'd padlocked his back wheel to mine and secured both to the metal cycle rack. I free his machine and I stand back with a 'there, that wasn't so bad, was it?' expression. He mounts up and with an ominous, rumbling grunt, like the noise an elephant makes when feeding, pedals away. 'Sorry,' I shout at the disappearing mountain. Without turning, he waves a hand the size of a shovel.

I have a warm feeling; instinctively I know I've made another friend. Relieved to have been spared I mount up and set off to take some photos of the Bullring, Birmingham's iconic shopping centre - then I notice that the bike has a pronounced wobble and the rear brake won't work. The big spindle that holds the back wheel on is missing. It's one of those quick-release jobbies that has obviously been quickly released by a local moron. It is also rather a crucial part of the machine because without it there is a danger of total collapse - which could easily result in unwelcome damage to my undercarriage.

I soon discover that cycling is not classed as a sport, at least here in central

Birmingham. I visit a number of sport shops in the city centre but none of them stock bicycle spares. If I'd have needed socks, I had the choice of approximately a billion. Raincoat? No problem - there's plenty of them, and non-sports trainers that start at sixty quid and progress up from there. I say 'non-sports' because at that price you'd want to frame and display them in a subtly-lit cabinet, not gallivant around a muddy field.

One particular sports shop is on the first floor. This necessitates my hauling the bike up an escalator in a shopping centre – to the surprise of one or two local browsers. I enter a well-known trendy sports store and stand looking around gormlessly until I'm rescued by a small lady with a local accent and wearing a flowery smock. She stops hoovering long enough to tell me the discouraging news that the nearest bike shop is in Selly Oak, two bus-rides and forty-five minutes distant. Then suddenly, with a big smile and a clap of her hands, she remembers another shop about twenty minutes' walk away. I thank her profusely, then she restarts her vacuum cleaner and disappears back within the forest of brightly-coloured clothing.

It is towards this actual cycle shop I push my wobbling apparatus. I am seeing rather more of our second city than I'd envisaged. Eventually I happen upon said emporium. It is single-fronted and rather grimy on a heretofore undeveloped street, in an undeveloped neighbourhood. Can you picture it? It's the sort of street that would have thrived in Victorian times but has been superseded by in-city Bullrings and out-of-town shopping complexes supplying Far-Eastern fabricated goods for those that want something cheap and disposable. The cycle shop is now considered niche, I suppose, a quaint oddity in an area ripe for flattening.

The bloke who runs the shop can't be described as quaint. He is a fit, tanned Australian guy with wiry muscles and curly blond hair - the sort of person you'd see jousting with fresh-water crocodiles in a Queensland wildlife documentary. He is also visibly distressed at the appalling condition of my bike. I have to say that surrounded by all that gleaming chrome it does look a bit like the poor relation. I assure him that I have allowed it to 'weather' so that there's less chance of it being stolen - and on that point he is forced to agree. I'm unconcerned about our appearance. Being a boater, dressing like an unsuccessful Womble, we're used to dirty looks.

While he attends to my bike, I stand self-consciously with bits of excess flesh poking out of my Lycra shorts, clutching my muddy, almost-blue helmet, trying to look like a proper sportsman. Repair completed, he follows me to the door, wishes me good luck, then turns 'open' to 'closed' and dashes off, presumably for a beer and a barby.

I arrive home at speed on two wheels, £6.50 lighter. My wife is slightly anxious because I'm an hour and a half later than expected, but I have another (mini) adventure under my belt. By a stroke of luck, the sun is just crossing the yardarm as I heave my bike onto the roof, just in time for a glass of athletes' reviver.

14

The Grey City Rollers

... is a cycling club - or was. It was my idea, I admit it. We set it up in France and it comprised a group of foreign nationals. If there has ever been a less successful cycling club in the world, ever, I would be fascinated to hear about it.

The 'Grey City' is St. Jean de Losne, in Burgundy, France where we lived for a while. The Rollers can refer to either the bicycles or those who ride them - a motley assortment of oddly-shaped people draped over steel frames. Ironmongery (or steelmongery, or even aluminiumongery?) strains under the weighty onslaught of mature folk who've partaken of too many cakes or too much wine, or both. I include myself here. Don't think I'm merely taking the piss out of everybody else - no, I'm very much part of this 'great' debate.

Notice the considered use of the word 'great.' It's very appropriate. It rhymes with 'ate,' contains the word 'eat' and signifies something substantial. In my case, that's me. It isn't difficult to notice that a number of us are rather on the porky side. Many of the folks who share my burden are nice people and they are my friends. Ultimately, I don't want to see them explode. But how to encourage them to exercise a bit without being insulting or patronising? The only way to do it, I thought, was to focus on me and see if I could get them to follow.

I'm not massively overweight, just moderately so. I even contemplate eating more baguette and butter to try and attain a flabbier starting point for my master plan. But then I look in the mirror and realize I don't need to. I am past the stage where I can simply pull my tummy in. In fact, when I try, a lump of spare flesh flops out somewhere else. 'Big-boned,' my friend terms it. He's being polite; I'm in need of an overhaul.

I tentatively ask my friends what they think about starting a cycling club. I'm wearing a tight t-shirt to emphasize my heftiness. I tell them I'm going to try and lose a few pounds. No time like the present, I suggest, but it's easier to embark on something like this with friends. Various nods and murmurs of agreement ... I propose we call the club, *The Grey City Rollers.* There are more enthusiastic noises so I press on and tell them that eventually the club will be open to everyone, but we will be founder members - we who share the pain of living in a dark place, namely a boat.

St. Jean de Losne is grey of colour but not of spirit, particularly during the summer months when the town thrives around the boating community and the number of residential boaters is swelled by summer visitors. Happy, sunburned specimens land among us wearing shorts and t-shirts. Some of them wish they'd paid less attention to the lager and takeaways over the winter. Perhaps they'll see us boating residents gliding around the streets like a parade of sylph-like deities and wish to join the fitness tsunami. This could be big ...

Anyhow, for now my friends agree that getting out there on bicycles is a good idea. I already cycle a bit so was relatively accomplished, at least in the eyes of some. One chap, a non-cyclist sitting on his boat drinking a cool beer, commented, 'I'll follow progress closely. After all, some club members are a number of stone over ideal and haven't ridden a bike for three decades.'

We're all bombarded with fitness regimes. Some of our number are Antipodean. These southern lands provide the blizzard of fitness experts (blonde, pearlescent teeth, spray-on leotards, four bronzed limbs) who skip about on a beach in the name of longevity, while twelve thousand miles away, in sleet-wracked Britain, thousands of porkers leap up and down in front of their TVs on a miserable January morning, curtains closed.

To encourage participation, I suggest that we go as slowly as the slowest person. That way nobody needs to feel overawed or inadequate. After all, if they are like me, there are plenty of other areas where they can feel inadequate.

The local topography is flat. Flat as a pancake, actually. We're in a large, low-lying basin stretching from Dijon 30 kms north-west to the Jura mountains to our east and, beyond that, Switzerland. The geography is why the summer temperatures can be stifling and winter can see minus double figures. It comes under the umbrella term of 'continental climate.' Umbrella. See what I did there? Summer feels like Death Valley, winter like the Siberian Steppes. As you'll realize, both extremes are less than ideal for a herd of plump cyclists.

On the plus side, the roads are quiet and of good surface, plus there's the option of the towpath running alongside the River Saone which passes north / south through St. Jean. The towpath is smooth and asphalt. The only slight concern is the proximity of the river should one of our number lose concentration while looking around for a cake shop. Then there are the local canal towpaths - the Bourgogne running up to Dijon and the Rhone au Rhin to the mighty Rhine, 140 miles east. Hang on, getting carried away. Something more modest to start with, I think.

Fortuitously, St. Jean also has its own Pompiers, the first response service for fire and medical emergencies. Professional help will never be far away, particularly the distances we plan to travel! So, the number one job at the start of our venture is to put Les Pompiers on speed-dial.

We plan the first trip with meticulous care. We choose a day when the weather promises to be neither sweltering nor freezing, with a light breeze. Wind is the enemy of super athletes. It's even more an enemy of less-than-super athletes, like us - largely to do with wind resistance (can I say 'largely'?). We scan the press to ensure there are no chocolate shops with half-price sales on and no cheese festivals within twenty miles. Right. No excuse for people to drop out. Green light!

Bicycles are procured. Some bikes come with the boats people had bought, a couple are borrowed; one chap even purchases one brand-new from the supermarket, such is his optimism. The day dawns. Mechanical checks are temporarily postponed as the biggest task commences; namely, the attachment of a bewildering collection of orthopaedic accessories to ankles, knees, elbows and any other part of the anatomy that needs support. Liniment is rubbed on, and first aid kits topped up. One person has a first aid haversack, required to cater for multiple age-related ailments. Tyres are pumped to bursting, chains oiled, brakes checked and off we go. As we wobble towards the town's boundary, I wonder whether we are actually going fast enough to require brakes!

There are seven of us, a good turnout for our first adventure. The route I've planned is a conservative one, a rotund six-kilometer plod. First leg: to the nearest village by road, then turn left for a spell before joining the riverside path for the gentle return to base camp. Things go splendidly for the first half hour; banter aplenty and nobody seems in undue distress. There is a peculiar whiff in the air. It's a chemical smell, but somehow reassuring. We narrow it down to over-heating liniment, and just accept that it as an occupational hazard associated with ageing fitness gurus.

But disaster strikes as we reach the village of Esbarres (pronounced prophetically, 'A Bar'). The village shop is open and a vote taken to stop and refuel. In fact, it isn't even a vote; it's more like a tectonic shift. Two members peel off the peloton and sit down outside the café. We've travelled only a conservative two kilometers, roughly the same distance you'd walk round a supermarket doing your weekly shop. The 'rebel two' are swiftly joined by the rest of us as we make ourselves comfortable outside the café under parasols in the village square. We overflow chairs that are barely up to their task. They're those little cast-iron seats, designed by Tarquin or Felicity to be used in minute city centre courtyard gardens, bijou set-ups to suit the upwardly mobile. What they're not designed to be is comfortable. Fortunately some of us are wearing padded shorts. So diminutive are the chairs that they look like stunted four-legged shooting sticks below our substantial posteriors. But comfort is not of primary concern when there are goodies on offer.

Considering the purpose of our outing - namely increased fitness - there doesn't seem to be a great desire to opt for the healthy options (not that there are many). Instead, we end up with a table full of double espressos, local liqueur chasers and an assortment of huge cakes, all ordered by pointing and sign language. Despite not speaking the native tongue, it's amazing how well you can communicate when you're greedy enough.

There are contented mutterings as we tuck into our well-earned treats. We sound like a herd of Gloucestershire Old Spots cheerfully munching their way through a field of snacks. If we'd each been teetering on the edge of a cardiac cliff at the start of the day, by the time we've cleared the shop out of everything unhealthy, well, let's just say my finger is twitching over the speed-dial button.

After a (very) short debate, the decision is taken to return home the way we've come rather than do the full circuit. So, we strap in and mount up - with a series of grunts and groans. We took rather longer to get home, unbelievably. In fact, we'd have been quicker walking. But that would have been contrary to our cycling club's constitution (if we'd had one).

Conversation is muted on the return journey as we concentrate on not dying.

But the day is sunny and the breeze light, and acres of puce flesh begin to turn a slightly deeper shade of pink. I did wonder whether we should have taken out travel insurance. I did have a brief look but couldn't immediately spot a *'meander'* policy designed for late-middle-aged wobblers. Should have looked for life insurance, perhaps?

As it turned out, I'd misread the map during the planning stages. There is a road towards the river from the village but no access to the towpath without going a further five kilometers downstream to find a bridge with access to the cycleway. That would have meant a round trip of nearer fifteen kilometers rather than the planned six. Those extra nine could have proved a bridge too far for most of us. But, thankfully, the fates intervene and I am able to record the inaugural outing of the Grey City Rollers in the annals thus: *Went to the nearest village and back with an enormous pit-stop half-way.*

On the second outing there were three of us. On the third, just me. Our club's annals are not extensive. A single page in history. Three weeks after the fanfares, it was all over.

Footnote: Our first (and basically only) excursion has gone down in folklore hereabouts. The café owner who serviced our needs on that first trip thought all his birthdays had come at once. So delighted was he at the scale of his unexpected takings, he installed a plaque on the shop front. We didn't really understand what it said, but think it translates something like, **'Pleasing to sponsor of the large English cycling people group.'** We believe it's a compliment. Whatever, he and his wife are probably still on holiday from the proceeds of our gluttony. In addition, local people who live along the route tell stories of a group of multi-coloured monsters moving at a similar speed to the snails they are so fond of.

Further footnote: The following month, there were five bicycles *'free to a good home'* in the local rag. For collection only.

15

Bikes and Boats

Towpaths are a great way to get around. As a rule, they are pretty level, often with a good surface. They connect towns and cities with fascinating bits in between. We ride on and adjacent to 200-year-old engineering, a fascinating slice of our industrial heritage. Industrial no more, of course; these days it's primarily leisure boats, an increasing number being used as an alternative or 'cheap' place to live.

It's not totally flat, of course. We have locks to cope with, sometimes a series of locks known as a flight or, where they connect directly one to another, a staircase. One particular flight of locks is a monster – the Devizes Flight, the top of which, as the name suggests, is in Devizes, Wiltshire. It links the Vale of Pewsey down towards the valley of the River Avon. The whole flight spans two and a half miles and twenty-nine locks but, most importantly for the cyclist, about 240 feet down and back up. It's a pretty steep hill. The Devizes Flight incorporates a series of sixteen consecutive locks known as the Caen Hill Flight. I had just completed the return trip and was standing at the top preparing to photograph engineer John Rennie's masterpiece of waterways history when a lady appeared next to me and said, 'What an astonishing piece of engineering.'

'Why, thank you,' I replied, trying to sound as humble as possible. 'I do try and keep myself in shape.'

She mumbled something and moved on. From which ever angle one looks, the Caen Hill Flight is a mighty impressive achievement. Looking from top or bottom, the lock-gates are perfectly aligned - almost impossibly so. From the air you see how the locks and their attendant side-pounds work to conserve water.

What's nice about the towpaths is that they connect lovely places. You can ride in safety through some magnificent countryside, taking in the odd hostelry along the way. Just by way of example, Devizes is a delightful market town home to, among other things, Wadworth 6X beer. Twenty-odd miles west is Bath in Somerset with stunning Pultney Bridge over the Avon, in addition to the Roman Baths and the Royal Crescent. The last two are a bit rich for me, but it's a great place to mooch around, particularly early morning when the hawkers and usurers are still abed. A couple of (relatively) easy hours between the two on a bike in a golden land. What's not to like?

It was in the aforementioned Vale of Pewsey that I cursed the general demise of the local shop. We had just cruised our boat from Pewsey to Alton Barnes, a distance of roughly five miles. It's very rural and I was looking forward to going to the shop which was advertised in our waterways guide – a reasonably recent edition, I might add. Rucksack on, off I went on my bike. I asked a bloke painting a window of a house where I might find the shop. 'Here,' he said. 'This was it. I've just shut it down after I was robbed again. Not worth the hassle. Nearest shop is over yon rise in Pewsey.'

I told him we'd just come from Pewsey, to which he replied, 'Ay, well.' Which I presumed meant 'Tough luck, you're off back there again.' I set off up yon rise, which became yon substantial hill, which in turn became a series of yon substantial hills. Very attractive rolling countryside, I must say, but cresting each rise I expected to see my destination laid out before me. However, unlike the canal, which followed a reasonably direct route, on the flat too, the road seemed to ignore every bit of level ground in Wiltshire. Of course, if I'd known the ride would have been so arduous, I would have gone down the canal towpath; but once you've gone part way on the road you tend to keep going.

When I finally got there, I collapsed in the 'mother and toddler' parking spot to get my breath back. I was trying to get shopping for three days but had to be circumspect with the weight or I might not even get back. I figured out that one sprout per day should be enough. Inexplicably, I returned by the same road rather than the towpath. By taking the road less travelled, and because I'd got some lamb chops to go with my sprouts, I reckoned I was being a mutton for punishment.

The variety of the seasons is wonderful too. Winter brings its own challenges, particularly when you have dodgy extremities. Spring is for new life when flowers hail the sun and birds sing their hearts out in search of a pal. Summer, when the contrasts are greatest, the shadows beneath the trees are darkest as foliage thickens and dry grass shimmers silver under the brightest sun. Autumn, my favourite, when nature is somehow at its quietest before the winds of winter blow away the year's husk. I didn't used to notice all this while stuck in a series of traffic jams. I can look around now rather than focus on the rear end in front.

$$* * *$$

On the continent I cycled many miles (or kilometers - there's more of them, so it sounds further). The Canal du Bourgogne and the Canal du Centre in Burgundy are home to leviathan hotel boats, floating monsters that fit tightly into the forty by five metre locks. Many of the guests pay big money to be wined and dined in five-star opulence while cruising through magnificent scenery. They stop off to visit some wonderful chateaux, vineyards and towns en route (bit of French crept in there!). Commercial boats on the canals are restricted in size to the dimensions of the locks. River cruise boats are much bigger, and can be more than three times the size.

Occasionally, while cycling I would come across the inmates of one of these hotel boats, and it could be an alarming experience. The poor tourists, a proportion of whom are substantial American specimens, get shoved off the boats (willingly, presumably) after breakfast to cycle down the towpath to the next port of call - to work up an appetite for lunch. To be frank, some of them look better suited to eating than cycling but it doesn't deter them.

They are invariably enthusiastic and chatty. I like Americans, at least the ones I encounter here on holiday. They are pleasant, fun people who cycle at a conservative pace – even by my standards. They make me look speedy - which is not easy to do. When I pass a line of them on my bike they often call an individual greeting along the lines of: *'Gooood mornin,'* splutter, *'ya have a good one now,'* wheeze, *'gee, it's a fiiine day,'* hack/splutter ... and so on.

* * *

We hadn't been in Holland long when Jan was gifted a bike. Our land-based neighbours saw her battling back from the shops on foot one day with a couple of heavy carrier bags. They asked why Jan didn't follow the example of a large proportion of Dutch people and use a bike for shopping. Many have panniers either side and a rack over the rear wheel. When they're not transporting children around, they can take a fair weight of shopping. Well, the answer was we hadn't got round to buying one. In fact, there were more important considerations - installing a lavatory on the boat, for example. The following morning, we found a bicycle on our front deck - a generous gift from our neighbour / friends. That bike stayed with us for ten years. It accompanied us all the way to France in a rack I installed on the rear deck. It wasn't the most modern piece of equipment, but for Jan to potter about on it was ideal.

I borrowed my friend's bike one day to go and pick up our car. A couple of days previously I'd driven our antediluvian Volvo to retrieve the boat, which we'd had to abandon having broken down - long story! Anyhow, I was riding along at a decent pace when I was passed by a ten-year-old girl perched on what looked like a sit-up-and-beg boneshaker. She was talking on the phone, her coat and hair streaming and flapping about behind her. These modern Dutch bikes are higher tech than they appear. I was riding a multi-gear mountain bike which was obviously built for adventure rather than progress (though why my friend had a mountain bike in the flattest country in the world, I'm not sure). I would never see the young girl again, would never be the butt of her speedy scorn, so allowed her to zoom off into the distance while I pretended not to feel inadequate. It was a sobering experience, if rather different to the one I had riding my step-daughter's bike a few years later. Oh, Lord, the jogger. He was somebody I might see again, which is why I changed my appearance by growing a beard and wearing a frock with tights underneath, which seems to be the fashion these days.

Jan and I were basically strangers in a provincial, church-going Dutch town; complete strangers till we got to know a few people. Jan went for a cycle one Sunday morning to get some exercise. It was winter so she was well wrapped up. Being Sunday, virtually the whole town was in one of the numerous churches dotted about the place, so when she stopped to rest on a bench she was totally alone. Until a motorcyclist pulled up. Over the course of the following few minutes he removed various items of winter clothing and his helmet and silk scarf. Finally free to speak, he asked Jan directions to a particular address, first in Dutch then, having met a blank wall, in English.

'No idea,' said Jan. 'I don't live here.'

The man, muttering furiously, redressed himself and went in search of somebody who wasn't a complete halfwit! Jan and I had a good chortle over that at Sunday brunch.

* * *

Back in France, we almost lost Jan's bike twice in a place called Migennes. First, she left it against the wall of the town's main market while she went to the loo, which in itself didn't go well. In fact, 'went to the loo' doesn't begin to describe the lavatorial pickle she got herself in. She managed to enter a fully-automated public lavatory mid-cycle. So, rather than having a pleasant, relieving experience, she got caught up in the flush / cleaning procedure, which took place in complete darkness. She emerged into to sunlight to face a queue of surprised locals waiting in line for the loo. She was fraught and drenched from head to foot with a bag full of soggy vegetables. When she went to retrieve her bike to make a damp retreat, she couldn't find it, despite making two complete laps of the market hall. Turns out a basket-seller had built a wall of baskets in front of her bike. Much to the angst of said basket-trader, a large portion of his rattan wall collapsed all over the cobbles as Jan,

63

in a state of some agitation, extricated her machine.

The same night her bike was taken from the rear deck of our boat. However, it appears that the thief was of discerning taste because we found it not ten yards away behind some folded-up trestle tables. Seems that whoever it was didn't want to be associated with Jan's faithful old cycle. I have to agree that it looked a bit mottled but it suited our needs and we finally said goodbye to it after ten faithful years when we included it in the sale of the boat - in fact, it probably clinched the deal.

16

River Runs

S ome of my favourite cycling memories are my rides on the banks of the wonderful River Loire. The river used to be navigated as part of the Route Bourbonnais, a four-canal north / south commercial waterway connecting Châlons-sur-Saône, on the River Saone, and St Mammes on the River Seine near Paris, thereby completing an inland waterway link between the Mediterranean and all points north. The Loire section of the route between Digoin and Briare was eventually replaced by the Canal lateral a la Loire which, as the name suggests, runs alongside the course of the river. The river was deemed too fierce in winter and unpredictably shallow in summer for navigation.

Anyhow, we were cruising our barge along that canal and got our first sight of the mighty river near Digoin. It gave me goosebumps. The Loire is not necessarily mighty in the same way the Amazon or Indus is, but it's an iconic waterway and to me it certainly warrants the tag 'mighty.'

I would take regular rides along the nearby river towpath. Frankly, it's magical cycling. We were there during the summer, so the river was gentle and shallow. It is generally wide with many sandbanks, the larger ones tree-populated. Water gently oozes around these mid-stream islands, creating slow-motion whirlpools in shades of blues and grey. It's a magical slow-motion aqua-ballet; a natural kaleidoscope designed to mesmerise. At least it did me - I'm easily mesmerised.

Amidst this wonder I came across something somehow typical of France - a concrete bench sited to take advantage of the incredible vista across the iconic river. At least it would have been if there weren't a line of enormous bushes between the bench and the river. No little things these, either - they were many years old and had somehow escaped the hedge-trimmer's tackle. Twenty feet left or right the view was unobscured and magnificent but right here where it wasn't required, an unruly hedge.

Then I thought about it and raised a pithy question. What if the bench was recently added? Which led to more questions. To objectify my curiosity, the initial question was the trunk, ongoing supplementary ones the branches, so we ended up with a veritable canopy of enquiry! Was the bench installer myopic or did they have a weird sense of humour? Or had I got it all wrong? Perhaps the hedge was made up of particularly rare specimens which were meant to be the primary object of interest. They must have been pretty special bushes to usurp the River Loire. Had the course of the river recently altered? Did it used to flow twixt bench and bushes (there's a song here, I think)?

This conundrum was vexing me as I mounted up and rode on. Then I happened upon something equally extraordinary, which had least had a logical explanation - a slip of a man, leather-skinned and lean as a rake, dressed in shorts and t-shirt, running towards me along the towpath followed by a lady on a bicycle. His pace is steady and she is rumbling along quite contentedly in his wake. She's wearing a long woollen skirt over leather ankle boots, all topped with a cape on this warm day. The bike has four panniers, two either side of each wheel, and what looks like a bedroll strapped behind the seat. They pause for the man to take a drink and we start chatting. Despite my schoolboy French, I do pick up what they are up to.

He is 67 and in the process of running 369 kilometers alongside the Loire, accompanied by his wife. She is his support vehicle and the panniers contain spare clothes, a tent, water-bottles, etc. They are taking a fortnight over their trip, travelling roughly 25 kilometers a day in the most wonderful setting. 'Why?' I ask him. 'To keep fit', he tells me, 'and because we wanted a challenge. As we get older,' he says, 'we need to test ourselves from time to time.' That is some test, I tell him. He nods and smiles. 'Allez-y,' he says to his wife. And off they go.

* * *

Just occasionally, I see a flat-bottomed 'traditional' barge typical of the shallow river. They are wooden boats, known as sand barges, some with a mast and sail, some with a motor. Many of the moderate-sized barges have a cabin towards the stern. Historically, the river has been used as a commercial thoroughfare for centuries but gradually fell from favour with the advent of the railways. The wooden barges were built in Orleans and much of the trade was between there and Nantes, near the river's mouth. At one time the barges would carry river sand from Orleans to Nantes to be used in construction. That trip would take about eight days. Because it would take at least double that time to do the return trip, it was uneconomical so some boats would be broken up and also used in construction.

I've come across plenty of slim boats (think hollowed-out log with a square front), four or five meters in length with an outboard motor perched on the back. These remind me of the type of thing I rode on in Bangkok; rapid and exciting water-taxis, similar to the thing James Bond got chased by.

One other ride I undertook was with my mate Bill. He and his wife Rosemary were our travelling companions for three months in 2010. Bill borrowed my wife's bike (swamped it, actually) and we rode to Bellville Nuclear Power Station. This monstrous power plant was around two kilometers from our boats on the canal, but the closer we got the more imposing it became. The enormous amount of excess heat the plant generates is cooled by the waters of the Loire. It's a fizzing, bubbling monster that made our hair stand on end. We didn't want to linger too long and spent a couple of megawatts of energy cycling back up the hill to safety.

I look back on 2010 with special fondness because it was my last year of carefree cycling. The following year I would begin to feel the effects of arterial problems, though it wasn't officially diagnosed for another five years. From then, it became a bit of a battle - right up till recently when I got my electric bike. Thanks to Columbanus, that fabulous world has recently reopened. But, what a special set of memories I have of riding along the banks of the Loire. In my mind's eye, I see the weathered runner as elderly, but I'm getting up towards his age and, even though not in as good a shape as he was, still feel inspired to find new adventures or test myself, as he put it, on my bike.

* * *

My bike shares wonderful experiences with me, but occasionally we come across the harsh reality of what man has done to man. One early morning in Verdun in 2009, not another living thing stirred. As I rode around the sandstone town, my bike's wheels chattered over the cobbles like the restless spirit of a muted machine gun whispering from almost a century ago.

The Hell of Verdun was a battle where Germany's plan was to 'bleed France white.' It lasted 300 days; there were over 700,000 casualties (of whom 300,000 died), shared pretty equally between French and German troops. I had the ghosts of these poor souls for company that morning. They perished so we could be free. Every day of the battle around 1,000 people died. How on earth can mankind do that to each other?

I sat alone on the steps below the monument to victory in Verdun. Alongside me a waterfall of fountains started its chattering descent down marble steps to the River Meuse. To me, the waterfall is symbolic of both constant change and moving on. If I merely sat and contemplated what had gone on around here, I'd never come to terms with it. I am seeing what happened from the distance of time. The fountain always looks the same and is forever here, but at the same time it's constantly moving on. It reminds me that we have to keep moving.

Behind me Charlemagne (or Charles I) stands atop Verdun's victory monument, leaning on a broadsword. Either side at ground level sit two great guns. During the day the town bustles with locals and visitors, but the backdrop to any thought or movement is the vile battle - something you wish wasn't there, but always will be. We've all seen on TV pock-marked buildings - in Beirut or Bosnia, for example - appallingly barraged by gunfire. Likewise, here there's a bullet-riddled building where goodness knows what happened to those inside. It's a clean, tidy town today, but whatever is done they'll be unable to wipe away the memories.

Equally moving is riding round parts of Flanders and seeing the memorials to many more who died for us; particularly the Menen Gate at Ypres, an imposing memorial in a lovely town immortalising another patch of hell. You can't fail to notice the numerous small cemeteries dotted round the landscape, some with just a couple of dozen white gravestones or crosses, melded forever into tiny corners of Europe. We lived in continental Europe for ten years and were never far from the memories of the World Wars. I often cycled country lanes and in the peace and quiet came across little graveyards tucked away, remembered only by relatives and those who tend the graves. Countries fight and joust even today; not on the same scale, but sabres are regularly rattled and it feels like we're one psychopath from another disaster.

17

Two-wheeled SUV

How do you describe a bike that is one's sole mode of transport? It's used for shopping, leisure, emergencies and a means of parading a god-like figure before his adoring public. Well, some of that's true. The last bit is never planned, it just happens during the course of daily activities. A burden I must bear with humility. We're talking about my Dutch euro-potterer now, pre bat-bike days. It's adaptable, seamlessly changing between uses. A convertible? Well, I suppose so. There's no roof, is there?

Emergencies? There's one I can remember. Me and a Dutchman once rushed across a marina to rescue a man trapped underneath his boat. I cycled round at great pace but was beaten by the seventy-year-old Dutchman, who was on foot! He was fitter than he looked - despite being somewhat overweight. (I let him win. I'm like that - considerate of others' feelings).

Leisure and shopping? Sure, panniers and rucksack are adequate. But where it fell down was transporting heavier stuff; a dozen cartons of milk, for example, or a 20kg sack of coal. Not things you want in a bag on your back, at least for any distance. We had used taxis on occasion, but that somewhat compromised our independence (not to mention making a couple of bags of coal mighty expensive).

Anyhow, where all this preamble is leading is that I built a trailer for my bike. Yes, built. A pal gave me a couple of wheelchair wheels with their brackets. I have to admit to having been a bit nonplussed at first. Why the hell would I want a pair of wheels off a wheelchair? Did I look that unsteady? It was he who suggested I use them as the basis for a trailer. He'd spotted some pieces of plywood on our rear deck, leftovers from another of my failed projects. Actually, I'd got properly cheesed off with this one. I'd carefully cut and painted the boards to use as internal 'floorboards' for an inflatable dinghy I'd been given. They fitted OK but when I got out of the boat, having given them a trial run, I left yellow, foot-shaped splodges on the pontoon. The paint hadn't dried properly so I'd had to wait before I got back on the boat, not wanting to leave yellow-splodges on the carpets. The paint wasn't the best, you see; it turned out it wasn't keen on moisture. Anyway, in a bit of a temper I'd thrown the useless boards on the back deck the previous autumn. By now, they'd had plenty of time to dry out, ready for re-purposing; hence my mate came up with the idea of a trailer.

Round the back of the boatyard workshops is a big pile of redundant scrap metal. Included in the pile was a set of stainless steel hand-rails from a motor cruiser. A little bit was bent and twisted, but the vast majority looked pristine; in fact, it was. Turns out the boat owner had just spent multi-thousands of euros on new rails but squashed them by hitting the very first bridge he came to. Insurance job - chuck the old stuff on the scrap heap. Enter fatso on the scrounge. I dug out some scrap angle iron for the corners and I was ready to go.

The upshot is that I did fashion a trailer. Looked OK, too. I held the whole thing together by stainless steel bolts with dome heads (so nobody could scratch themselves on open-ended threads). I needed about forty small bolts which were nearly a euro a set from the local (rip-off) merchants. Couldn't complain, though - everything else was free / scrounged.

So, time for a test run. Two minor niggles. Firstly, it squeaked; secondly, it wobbled from side to side like me going too fast on the bat-bike or a caravan behind a car without an adequate stabilizer - just slower and much less attractive. My wife was following this first trial run so she could spot anything untoward. She nearly fell off laughing as I wobbled and squeaked toward the boulangerie. She giggled as I soldiered on with pride and defiance. But a little oil and another lump of stainless bolted on as a brace and it was quite serviceable.

So, by adding a trailer, I'd turned a thing used for sporting magnificence into something of actual practical use. Our very own two-wheeled SUV. Actually, it was four-wheeled now. I gave it a proper test by cycling to the supermarket for diesel. A pair of twenty-five litre drums of diesel is pretty weighty and, considering it sloshes around a bit, I just prayed that nothing went wrong travelling busy roads, including roundabouts.

Out of interest, I believed I was carrying fifty kilos of diesel, but in fact I wasn't. Diesel is more than ten percent lighter than water, so I was overestimating my capabilities. This is why you see diesel floating on water, making those nice kaleidoscopic patterns. Anyhow, on the roads I didn't travel too fast and got a few waves from motorists - some in greeting with an amused smile, the odd one more 'earthy' and along the lines of, 'What the bloody hell are you doing on a busy road on that death trap?'

I was back unloading my diesel when a man happened by in need of assistance. He saw me at work and zeroed in on me as someone practical, believing me the kind of chap who could turn his hand to anything (ahem). As I fiddled with my trailer, he obviously recognized a skilled engineer when he saw one. Whatever, he stopped and asked for my help. If there had been an Academy Award for mucking up a repair job I would, at the very least, have received a nomination.

His machine was laden with gear for what was obviously a prolonged trip. He looked a bit fraught as if he'd been pushing his bike for a while already. A man at the end of his rope, with a malfunctioning bike pump. His rear tyre was only half inflated, so he asked if I could pop some air in it. All he wanted was sufficient pressure so he could cycle to a shop to buy a new pump. It was a valve-type that I hadn't encountered previously but nevertheless I had a go. I tried a number of different nozzle adapters. Ten minutes later his tyre was completely flat.

Whatever I tried, the tyre would just not accept air. The man watched with increasing resignation as the recalcitrant tyre sat flaccidly on the concrete. I told him with some authority that his tyre was knackered, most likely the valve. Not sure he understood but he walked away with a resigned (to be polite) look, shoulders slumped as if he was burdened with life's troubles. There was a squeaky, rubbery sound as he wheeled his steed away and was lost to sight behind the toilet block.

'Is there no beginning to your talents?' asked my friend, as the sound of the deflated Frenchman faded away.

18

Plainly more than a Pylon

There is a joy being up high and looking down. I'm only a short chap so don't often get to see the tops of people's heads. Being on a hill with my binoculars I can see bald patches and double crowns galore. Bustling ant-like folk, both at work and play, skitter around the valley floor. Tiny vehicles zip to and fro. Then, scan up the hillside where horses, sheep and cows graze distant moors chaperoned by the occasional roe deer. Up on the tops, the same height as me, giant wind turbines have invaded and settled in the choicest locations, exhibitionists, visible to all. They suck the life out of the moors, feeding on an ever-present breeze. They are prominent and frankly pretty ugly, but they are here to stay. It took a while, but I have become somewhat immune; they are now part of the landscape.

One thing that does get on my wick is electricity pylons. I remember them going up hereabouts in the 1970s and they are scars on the land, to be sure. But somebody loves them - incredibly, there is a Pylon of the Month! I kid you not. I can scarcely believe this, but May 2021's pylon is just outside Oxford. According to the writer on the website *'Pylon of the Month'* (yes, there is one!) there's a good pub nearby so *'after a walk round the area it may be time for a pint and a pylon.'*

It gets weirder. April's pylon is near Milan, northern Italy. According to the write-up in *Pylon of the Month*, a man named Giangiacomo Feltrinelli was found dead at the bottom of it. He was a one-legged, 46-year-old chap who translated Doctor Zhivago after the manuscript had been smuggled out of Russia. He was therefore indirectly responsible for Boris Pasternak being awarded the Nobel Prize for literature in 1958. Anyhow, Mr Feltrinelli was apparently a bit of a left-wing activist and had allegedly been trying to blow the pylon up when he came to grief! According to his son, Feltrinelli was *"a difficult man devoted to a certain type of risk, together with a surprising form of irreverence that speakers of Yiddish [know] as 'chutzpah.'"* Could you make all this up? I couldn't.

Back in the real world, if you can ignore the man-made monstrosities that litter the landscape, it's really quite beautiful seen from on high. Around where I live, stone slate roofs protect century-old farmhouses from fierce Pennine weather. Reservoirs on the moors twinkle blue, reflecting the sky, while way down below the canal snakes green along the valley floor, reflecting the valley sides. Often the railway follows the course of the canal, because it takes the route less hilly, but here the railway is more than 120 feet below my feet as its course is through the Summit Tunnel. What amazes me is that the tunnel is 180 years old and still carries trains today, yet when they resurface a road it's knackered before your chips have gone cold.

The tunnel endures despite there being a huge accident and ensuing fire in 1984. A petrol-carrying train crashed in the tunnel and two of the thirteen tankers actually melted at over 1,500 degrees. Despite some of the bricks 'vitrifying and flowing like molten glass,' the tunnel withstood the blaze and was re-opened with minimal structural repair within a year. That is some testament to the tunnel builders.

The canal is even older than the railway. The original canal route was surveyed by James Brindley way back in 1766 but didn't open fully until 1804 (32 years after Brindley's death). Despite it being well over 200 years old, the Rochdale Canal still carries boats across the Pennines. The infrastructure, unsurprisingly, is showing its age in places.

Frankly, pioneering engineers, such as Brindley and Telford, were as-tonishing. Brindley was consulting engineer on the Bridgewater Canal which transported coal from the Duke of Bridgewater's mines at a hugely reduced cost compared to the horse and cart method, thereby helping fuel the industrial revolution. Brindley also oversaw the below-ground channels within the coal mines, an astonishing 46 miles of them. This even included an underground incline plane that connected two levels of the mine. Coal was transported on boats called 'Starvationers' - long, narrow craft, forerunners of the narrowboat. Why the name? They were built with extra-strong ribs to cope with the weight they carried, so they looked like the rib cage of a starving person.

As I stand on the hill and look way down, I'm standing on an old pack-horse route that would have been used to carry goods on horseback over the hills. I can't help but marvel at the imagination and skill of the canal engineers and builders of yesteryear. Years ago I wrote a long poem about our narrowboat days that included a reference to the kind of spot I now stand ...

> *A thousand trudging weary nags*
> *pulling heavy loads*
> *'cross windy, chilly Pennine hills*
> *on pitted rocky roads.*

I have a few favourite circuits which vary in length between six and twenty-one miles. I tackle different ones depending on local weather conditions and how knackered I feel. Each route has a climb with the reward of a view, and each involves a differing amount of canal towpath. My long loop includes Cragg Vale, known for being the longest continuous gradient in England. It's five and a half miles, or nine kilometers, with a rise of 970 feet. I've only tackled this downwards so far! Not sure the battery would last going uphill. (I realize that at twenty-one miles my 'long' route is a mere warm-up distance for better cyclists, but we do what we can - and it's about my present limit.)

It's a great ride down Cragg Vale, all the way from the fabulous moorland up top, through a steep-sided wooded vale to the valley below and the various modes of transport that link Todmorden and Halifax (road, canal, railway). Down here I join the Rochdale Canal. Turn right to Sowerby Bridge where it enters the Calder & Hebble Navigation or left all the way (about thirteen miles) home to Littleborough via Hebden Bridge and Todmorden. Nearly twenty miles beyond Littleborough is Manchester and the Bridgewater Canal. I'm in Mytholmroyd and ride the canal towpath all the way home from here.

I have driven this road for more than forty years. I first cycled this circular route more than forty-five years ago. I would have been riding my previously-mentioned Raleigh Olympus (duly repaired, having been squashed). The road snakes along the valley floor, sharing the space with the canal and River Calder. The towpath ride is particularly good because they've resurfaced much of it after a proportion of it was basically washed away in recent flooding. The River Calder can be a brute for flooding, as we found out to our cost numerous times when our shop in Todmorden submerged. Even on a sunny day, parts of the valley are gloomy because the sun doesn't penetrate the trees on steep valley sides.

There are communities of live-aboard boats scattered along the route. Some of the boats look in need of a repaint, after they've had a good wash. Boat living is considered a budget way of life but one wag said that living on a small boat is like being in prison with the additional threat of being drowned. You may know that we lived on boats for twelve years. When not cruising we were in a marina. Not sure I could cope with the conditions here, but there's a thriving community.

Having said that, it's all a question of degrees. To some people living in impressive, boxy modern houses in gated communities, those whose lives are governed by nail extensions and Range Rovers, the idea of living on any sort of canal boat is a nightmare. Even the most expensive, highly glossed boats housed in prestigious marinas would be a lowering of standards too precipitous to contemplate. Our boat was 'medium-good' and we lived in a decent marina with fabulous people. I have to confess to shuddering somewhat when we passed a fibreglass wreck that was obviously someone's home. I've no right to judge anyone, but it does make me consider what differing reasons make people choose a life on the canals.

For us, it was an exciting change of lifestyle when we thought Jan didn't have long to live. For some it may be a retirement dream, for others it may be for financial reasons. Some people are just free spirits who want to drift on life's current.

Things have changed since we started boating back in the early 2000s, no doubt about it. It's much busier, especially round 'honey-pot' sites like London or Bristol, for example. We looked for what we could get out of the experience, but now an increasing number look to what they can get out of the system. If you compare an inexpensive boat to a modest flat in London the difference is hundreds of thousands, so it's not surprising that people seek the cheaper option. If this means hopping from bridge to bridge every few days, it's a small price to pay.

In and around Hebden Bridge the canal is thriving and cycling it is a pleasure. Local residents have planted a ribbon of flowers between the towpath and the canal. Now this may be a way to deter boats mooring outside their property, but for me passing through it really is lovely. On the outskirts I pass a pub that used to belong to friends of ours, Bob and Rita. Sadly, they are both dead to cancer, Rita first. Whether running pubs and bars in smoky atmospheres had anything to do with it I can't say, but each time I cycle past I doff my cap and recall some fond memories.

Bob had his voice box removed not long before he died, so he struggled to communicate. In fact, he said (by writing it down for us) that people didn't really know how to engage with him because he couldn't talk. I found it sad that people seemed to be ignoring him because they hadn't the imagination to find a way to connect. He needed to communicate, as a therapy if nothing else, to remember and talk about Rita - of whom he was obviously enormously fond. Then Bob died, too, and we're left with a pub on which to focus our memories. I wonder how long the pub will last.

Passing the rear of the Picture House I remember going to 'An evening with Rick Wakeman.' A man after my own heart this, who enjoyed his ale and his curries till a number of heart-related episodes by the age of 25 prompted a change of behaviour! But the guy who played piano on David Bowie's *Life on Mars* will always be my play-list friend. This is lovely, you see ... memories wherever I look.

19

Bush Hats and Batteries

When I was a nipper we lived in a house that had a shrubbery. Sounds posh, eh? In essence it was a small patch of ground on a steep slope with a few bushes on it. I can assure you it was nothing like a Lancelot 'Capability' Brown creation. No, ours was like something you'd see at an abandoned coal mine, where stunted trees and bushes battle for survival in coal-spoil earth. But kids don't care as long as there's somewhere to play. I pestered Mum into buying me a bush hat, which was basically a camouflaged, floppy sun hat. I think I got the idea from the TV programme *Daktari* - remember that?

Pretending to be a covert assassin, I would crawl around the shrubbery in my hat, totally camouflaged from my unwitting targets. Never mind that I also wore red pants and yellow shirt - irrelevant. The hat did its job and I invariably completed my missions undetected. The unfortunate postman didn't know what hit him, nor the grey-suited man from Betterware with his boot-full of household must-haves. Unlike my real-life brothers-in-arms in the SAS, I didn't go as far as staying immobile for days on end or pooing into a plastic bag, but I was a pretty lethal killing machine nevertheless.

Roll on nearly sixty years and I'm still trying to pull the wool over people's eyes. These days I'm imitating an athlete atop my electric wobbler. In place of the bush hat, I wear a blue helmet over a nasty green top and 'Stanley Matthews' shorts. I actually met Mr Matthews a number of years ago and what a gentleman he was. He reached the pinnacle of his sport and I think he'd have been both dismayed and amused at my athletic deception while wearing his shorts.

In fact, not only am I impersonating an athlete through my attire, but Columbanus isn't even a 'proper' bike, as I'm frequently told by unassisted riders. But we live in a world of misconception and deception. Many of us pretend to be someone we're not by hiding behind a veneer, whether material, cerebral or technological. Similarly, many of us see something that's not there. Just because somebody is driving a decent car or wearing nice clothes doesn't make them happy. Mind you, until recently I wore 'basic' attire and drove a right old heap, where there was little room for envy. Pity, more likely! I can't possibly have appeared contented to anyone with an ounce of modern-world realism, but I was.

The thing about my e-bike is that I can get away with my slight deception. I can zoom up a hill, passing proper cyclists as I go. I don't actually hide the facts, I just don't mention them. Unless someone asks of course, then I tell them: "Yes, it's electric but I've got it turned off. You think these bulging quads are just for show?" By the time they've formulated a suitable insult, I've gone round the bend. Which rather sums it up.

When in battery mode, I do exaggerate the respiratory noises on occasion. Although I'm actually reasonably comfortable in cruise mode, I like to make it appear as if I'm on the ragged edge. As an unfortunate consequence, the proper cyclist feels even more inadequate when they're passed by someone sounding like Darth Vader's asthmatic uncle. But my search for that endorphin rhapsody is all-consuming, so other people's feelings are the least of my worries. Particularly when the motor genuinely won't work and I have to turn round and go back downhill.

The other thing that people assume is that I'm enjoying myself. Most of the time I am, but when I'm getting near the top of a longish climb I would happily swap places with most people, particularly if they're going past on a bus. I observe other cyclists and there's a 50:50 chance they will acknowledge me. Sometimes it's hard to spot - the lifting of a finger or the raise of an eyebrow. Let's be honest; you can't manically wave, can you? You'd be in the ditch. Not many people actually look to be enjoying it, though, either cycling or running. A lot of money is spent on equipment and clothing to end up looking miserable. The ultra-serious exerciser (not me) keeps a poker face and has total focus. There are two possible reasons for this:

1. They need to maintain their 'I'm-undoubtedly-fitter-than-you' image, or
2. The Fat-Bit they wear detects mirth and delivers an electric shock. Fun is not allowed!

(Difficult to tell with No. 2 sometimes because a grin and a grimace are close bedfellows.)

I tend to be sociable whether my targets want to reciprocate or not. It's often people of a similar age to me who enjoy a chat. Of course, that means stopping and it's often noticeable that both of us are glad of a breather. Plus, of course, folks my age tend to have time for a natter. Not long ago, I was up on top of the moors when, in the distance, I spotted a group of people wearing white robes and chanting. They were quite some way off and I didn't have my binoculars with me, so couldn't really make them out. There was a guy jogging towards me, so I asked him if he knew what was going on. Not a peep - no reaction whatsoever. He was in another world, one that included headphones (or buds these days) and that thousand-yard athletic stare. How can people be so oblivious to what's going on around them?

Turns out the chanters are a Christian religious sect who come up on the moors regularly. On subsequent occasions I've seen them rather closer up and they are all black people, some of whom are carrying crooks. I read that there are a number of white-robed Christian groups and as far as I'm concerned it's a fine way to pass an early morning hour. There's something slightly threatening about hooded white robes, crooks and chanting, but I spoke with a guy who had stopped and talked to one group; he said they were lovely, gentle folk out on the moors to pray, a threat to nobody.

But that wasn't the case in Barnsley (Yorkshire) recently. A similar group went out into the woods to chant and fell foul of the 'noise police' in nearby houses who claimed their Saturday lie-in was being compromised. This puts me in mind of those reports of city people who've migrated to the country only to complain bitterly about a noisy cockerel cock-a-doodle-dooing at daybreak, as they have done since time began. Perversely, the city dweller is oblivious to a moron singing *'Football's Coming Home'* through a kebab at 3.00 AM, but present them with a real animal behaving as evolution intended and there's a letter fired off to Environmental Health.

One benefit of advancing age is the freedom to think about things and look more closely - if you have a mind to, of course. The white-robe group reminded me that I'd recently seen a Christadelphian Hall close to where we live. There are plenty of religions or branches of religions, but this was a 'sect' I'd never heard of. So, I investigated and I'm not much the wiser. Christadelphians are described variously as 'a restorationist and millenarium Christian group who hold a view of biblical Unitarianism' or 'a non-trinitarian, millennial Christian group.' That's cleared that up then!

I turned my mind to how I could describe my cycling family while disguising the fact that I'm basically a half-baked blob. How about: 'Revolutionary, multi-shaped thrill seekers, frequently accused of obstructing the progress of idiots in charge of internal combustion engines'? Actually, that makes **too** much sense. While I'm on my next ride, I'll think of another which will include some quasi-Latin and a few 'isms.'

20

Get Your Kicks ...

M y local canal cycle path is Route 66, part of the Sustrans network. '66' runs from Manchester to Spurn Head, Yorkshire's Land's End. The route goes via Kingston upon Hull, a city I thought I'd never been to, but I have. It's Hull's alternative (Sunday) name. Sounds rather posher than just Hull.

The bits of Route 66 I've walked, boated and cycled over the years are largely a dozen miles east or west from home. Lovely territory along the valley floors between Pennine hills. On recent occasions I've taken my time and and have been able to see and learn a bit about things that have been within a stone's throw all my life.

One tidbit is that the last lock on the canal is lock 92, yet these days there are only 91. Locks 3 and 4 were merged in 1996 to form one deep lock at Tuel Lane in Sowerby Bridge. Known sometimes as 'the Everest of Canals,' the Rochdale Canal was the first of three trans-Pennine canals, the others being the Leeds-Liverpool and the Huddersfield. All of them, at times, are very rural and stunning.

Cycling is my preference these days but there are some tracks that even my dear old bike can't cope with, so I walk instead, particularly on Blackstone Edge where the tracks are little more than scars etched into the moors by sheep and walkers. I walk on gritstone, a name that sums up nicely the rough, harsh landscape. Gritty or not, the views are terrific - when there's no rain or fog. It's wild and open and you can feel like someone discovering it all for the first time. However, I must be at least the second person up here because of the Aiggin Stone, a four-feet high gritstone way-marker, thought to have been here for 600 years. It's by the side of a track that some think was originally a Roman road, latterly a packhorse trail. It goes straight over the hills from Littleborough to Yorkshire. Why on earth would anybody want to go to Yorkshire, particularly when it used to be even more primitive than it is today? A mystery historians still puzzle over - often over a pint in the nearby White House pub.

Also up here are channels, or water highways, that ship water between reservoirs. As required, this hilltop water is released to supply the canals and nearby towns down below. Warland Reservoir, for example, was constructed by the Rochdale Canal Company around 1827 to supply the Rochdale Canal. Warland is a Category A reservoir. *'Oh,'* I think to myself, *'that's nice - something prestigious on our doorstep.'* Well, not really. Category A means that it has the capacity to 'threaten life in the event of a failure.' As me and plenty of other people live below it, I would rather it was recategorized as a 'Category C', like my grandson's paddling pool, with the legend, 'Beware of the odd splash.'

Down at 'sea level,' way down in the valley, there's a little hamlet after which the reservoir was named. Warland is a tiny settlement right by the canal on the Lancashire- Yorkshire border. One lady who lived there in a cottage wanted her son to go to school in Yorkshire but the authorities said he must go in Lancashire because that's where her house was. Then she realized that her outside toilet was in Yorkshire. She appealed, and they got their wish - he went to school in Yorkshire. At least his back end did.

The route I ride home from Warland passes an old toll house with its fascinating scale of charges for passage over Calderbrook Road, which linked Todmorden and Littleborough (Yorkshire and Lancashire, in effect). The tolls are not straightforward either. They were determined by the width of wagon wheel. Six inches or over - 5 d (old pennies), graded inch by inch to 'less than 3 inches' - 9 d (the narrower the wheel the more damage to the road, I presume). 7d for a 'chaise', litter or hearse (posher vehicles). Unladen horse, mule or ass - 2 d. Ox, cow or neat cattle - ½ d. Calf, sheep, pig or lamb - ¼ d. (How things change - 1/4 d is about one tenth of a decimal penny). I must have driven and ridden past this tollhouse ten thousand times and not had the inclination to stop and look. Lucky you. Now I've taken the trouble, you've got the info for no effort!

What's 'neat' cattle, I hear you ask? Well, it's an obsolete term for cows or bulls, or a collection of same. So 'neat' cattle on the toll charges must be a collective of cows. Why the 'neat' cost should differ from charging single cow by single cow, I'm not sure.

The toll house is still lived in. Round the corner there's a plaque on the gate threatening anyone leaving it open be liable to a fine 'not exceeding forty shillings.' A modern addition, I think. Two quid for allowing their dog to escape? A generous price indeed.

From the summit of this particular road, I have access to a precipitous little track that climbs steeply off to the right before running a mile or so along the top of the valley side before returning, via another cliff, to the valley. For much of the time I'm separated from a near-vertical drop only by a flimsy fence. It's a harsh climb but I've a terrific view when I finally get to the top. It's taken a couple of drinks breaks, four deep-breath breaks and one pee stop. The latter was precautionary, one I thought prudent to take in case they had to load me into an ambulance. Need to preserve my dignity. What's left of it.

To my right, part way down the slope, is one of the circular, stone-built ventilation shafts that service the Summit railway tunnel through the hill below. I have a photo taken from the opposite side of the valley showing fire and black smoke pouring from the shaft after the train crash I mentioned earlier. It's astonishing. The top of the shaft is more than 30 meters below me, but the flames would have burned higher than where I stand. Boy, that's some fire.

Up to my left a grove of wind turbines, their blades lazily turning. But they're quiet, trying to blend in. A little further along I look straight ahead to the east to see, clinging to the hillside, Todmorden Golf Club where I spent many frustrated hours. In fact, I dislodged so much turf with my manic hacking that the hillside has quite a different profile than when I'd started thirty-five years previously. I gave up golf many years ago but my brother is still rearranging the landscape.

The track deteriorates, to exactly a condition you'd expect in territory where only animals have the dim-wittedness to roam. What's the term for something worse than a track? Not sure, but it's more than a path. In fact, parts of it are nearly as bad the main road outside the junior school in town. I have to go through a farm gate that opens 'the wrong way' - in other words towards me from the left. It swings out over a muddy stream so there's nowhere for me to stand. I have to leave the bike some way back then prop the gate open, retrieve the bike and proceed through. By the time I'm free and clear I've aged somewhat and its tea-time. So I press on determinedly,

I'm still high up but thankfully the road improves and I drop down on tarmac after a nervy 'Tour de France' descent. I emerge near a garden centre where I recently bought a couple of bags of compost and a pair of socks. Doesn't everyone seem to be diversifying these days?

I look up to where I've come from. I've just cycled the shape of a large lay-by, but set on its side at 45 degrees, and there's no way I would ever have been up there without Columbanus. In truth, he hasn't let me down at all yet, apart from the flat tyre when I first got him. Oh, and the occasion he lost concentration on a rubbly road and tipped me off. Thankfully it wasn't a full-bloodied crash, more of a graceful tumble sideways. I rolled, like an uncontrolled green beetle, through tussocky moorland grass before coming to rest in a patch of reeds. It was more like a graceful Tai Chi move performed at Grandma's Zumba class than a spectacular wipe-out. I'm not built for major wipe-outs these days.

II

Part Two

The Howgill Fells

21

The Howgill Fells

B etween the Lake District and the Yorkshire Dales lies a slice of heaven. It's a peaceful, remote land, untroubled by the manic world beyond. Ewes, with their unbearably cute lambs, share the landscape with fell ponies, red squirrels, a myriad of birdlife and Pendragon's castle. In addition, a branch of my family that has moved here to begin a new life. They are near a village and range of fells of which I had never previously heard – Ravenstonedale and the Howgills, respectively. But I will get to know them.

Into this garden of Eden comes a chap who's eaten too many pies. A man attempting to reverse the effects of fifty years of dreadful diet. And boy, does any physical shortcoming get found out in these hills. I venture out for my first foray on foot in the company of the dog. Later, it'll be just me on my bike. Half an hour into my first outing, I'm a wreck. Somehow it's all uphill. Even the downslopes are uphill! I'm used to living next to a football field in a bungalow, and pottering around either of these is poor preparation for a series of precipitous fells. And, I have to be honest here, I haven't actually left the road yet!

My start point is at 940 feet and I climb another 400 or so to where I reach the highest point of this single ribbon of tarmac. Along the road there are periodic passing places and occasional solid ground exits onto the fells. These are used by quad bike hill farmers tending their flocks. Either side of the road, which is only about three meters wide, runs a small, damp ditch so you have to pay attention when cycling or in a vehicle or you could get trapped at a boggy angle. In my brief experience, it's unusual to meet another road user. Apart from sheep, that is, and they generally amble off out of the way.

The fells rise massively to each side and before me. The highest point in the Howgill Fells is The Calf at 2,218 feet. That's nearly a thousand feet above where I'm already in a state of some distress! The air where I am, at 1,345 feet, is chill and clear. I have found my new favourite spot. The road does extend down beyond this crest for half a mile or so. It ends in an isolated farm. Beyond there, the only onward access is via bridleway or on a quad bike (or on foot) over the fells.

When my heart stops thumping, there's a silence so intense it quietly hisses. That is, until the cry of a curlew fractures the stillness, ending in that familiar rippling trill. They fly close by sometimes, often in pairs, pointing the way with their familiar curved bill. A melody synonymous with the stunning landscape that wraps me up and holds me spellbound. It's not often I just want to stand and stare, to soak up my surroundings and never leave. But I'm rooted. Even the dog sits still and absorbs nature's theatre.

From my crest I can see many miles as the first rays of the sun turn the hill tips auburn. The colours develop through vibrant red / brown / orange - the fells on fire. But it's a fleeting look lasting a few precious moments while the sun peers through a low-level veil as it crests a distant moor. Within minutes the light is bright and the hills turn gold. I've had a go, but to be honest I haven't sufficient words.

* * *

We are staying in a property called The Green, about a mile south of Raven-stonedale village in the Howgill Fells. We're about five miles from Kirkby Stephen. The property is owned by my step-daughter Carly and partner Richard. They are a terrific couple at the height of their powers. The Green is set in a couple of peaceful acres and the whole property comprises the owner's ex-farmhouse and a large separate building converted into three holiday apartments. We're staying in one of these. We're also working on them. We're on a working holiday, if there is such a thing. Lots of banging in of nails and screwing in of screws to ready the accommodation for their first guests.

The apartments were originally set up 12 years ago by the previous owners and they still hold a five-star rating. Judging by the level of equipment and finish, I find it hard to imagine they could have made a profit on the sale; it must have cost a fortune to set up. For example, there is a HUGE underfloor heating set-up starting forty yards from the accommodation block with underground pipes in the garden. What looks like many hundred yards of big-bore pipework connect to two large refrigeration / compressor units in the garage, then on to three separate systems (one for each letting unit) with separate and thermostatically controlled zones in each unit, upstairs and down. A very large scale set-up - not cheap to install and not that cheap to run either, I suspect. During this chilly April, the warm floors are a real boon for my diabetic feet. It's comforting to soothe my feet on a warm dog on a chilly evening.

Each unit has all the mod cons and a few extras besides. I must say they are really nice. What Carly is doing is updating equipment, soft furnishings and decor. She is giving them a throroughly modern feel. Imagine upgrading one house and tripling it?! This is where we come in. Carly has given me a list of tasks that reads like the King James Bible - lots of chapters with plenty of verses. Holy Moses.

Just out of interest, our hosts are not married. Carly is my step-daughter, so what does that make Richard? Step-partner-in-law? They have provided the world with two delightful lads, two rays of sunshine that brighten even the darkest Cumbrian day. They have worked incredibly hard to get here and now stand on the end of their springboard ready to leap into their new life.

Richard has trained as a Mountain Leader. He leads groups on hikes and walks on the hills and fells throughout the UK. Locally he is termed 'Crag Rat,' the friendly colloquialism for a mountaineer.He and his clients trek the moors, sometimes many miles. He teaches them survival and navigation skills and makes a good living out of something he loves with a passion, using leg muscles, power and brawn. I, meanwhile, use my brain, imagination and creativity to write articles and books and am considerably less successful!

The first day of our working visit is 4th April 2021. It's the start of a special time spent with family in a wonderful place. Our self-contained apartment is across the yard, so during these virus-hit times we are comfortable and well distanced. Anybody who comes here for a holiday in the future is in for a treat.

Exactly twelve years ago, coinciding with the day of our arrival in Cumbria, we set off on our boat from central Netherlands bound for Burgundy, central France. An 'on this day' photograph flashed up on my phone. It shows a fishing boat leaving harbour in a little Dutch town called Hardewijk (pronounced hardyvike) on the shores of the Ijsselmeer, which was formerly called the Zuider Zee. Numerous long and circular hooped nets, called Fyke nets, hang from the rear of the boat. They are designed to catch eels, known as paling (pronounced parling), a staple in The Netherlands. That photograph marked the start of a memorable six-month adventure for us. It feels like one branch of our family is embarking on their own wonderful odyssey.

As I say, we're here to work (partly).

'Should I bring my tools?' I asked my stepdaughter during the planning stage.

'No, no, no. Goodness, please don't.' Lengthy pause. 'You can use Richard's.'

We performed tasks of which they were quite capable but short of time. Between my wife and I, plenty of DIY, ironing, sorting and child-minding. But we made time for us, too. My very first walk amazed me as you'll have gathered by my initial impressions. There is so much to see and experience, including some amazing bike rides.

22

By Gum, it's chilly

Today I let Columbanus loose on the fells; hopefully, my trusty steed will earn his spurs. He's been up plenty of hills before, but there's always been somebody within shouting distance if either of us suffered a mishap. Even up on top of the Pennines, where it feels pretty remote in places, there would be somebody along 'in due course' to administer first aid, mechanical or physical. Or, God forbid, last aid. Except, of course, if it's chucking it down when neither we nor anyone else would be there. It gets a bit fierce on the tops.

Today we're going to be pretty isolated. Leaving the house, we cross a cattle grid then a stone bridge over a chattering beck. There's about a quarter of a mile of uphill gravelly track before we're finally on to a bitumen road, itself only a scant four paces wide. We turn left, away from the village, towards the high fells and a few isolated farms. Immediately, it's steeply uphill before it levels out somewhat to be just mildly uphill. Even in lowest gear the steepest bits are a struggle. The general topography is basically rolling hills, mainly uphill while heading south, which we are.

There's also a biting south-easterly wind blowing. Wind is the enemy of the cyclist, particularly a fat one going uphill. To reach the point I did on foot yesterday, there are basically three sharp rises, each a few hundred yards long. The third is the steepest. At one point, on a steep bend, there are skid marks on the road where vehicles have struggled for traction. Every fifty yards or so is a yellow grit bin, supplied by the council. These bins are pirated by the sheep searching out the salt. I even saw one sheep standing fully inside a bin, having already opened the lid!

On the final ascent, about fifty yards up this stretch, I come to a grinding halt by the first such bin and use it as a seat. My thighs are like jelly and burning. I'm in some discomfort when, through my tears, I see four people coming down the hill towards me. Leading the party is an elderly lady, muffled up so just her eyes are visible. She's wearing a thick coat, gloves, scarf and hat. And she's riding a mobility scooter! No ordinary 'let's nip down the shops' type scooter either. This is the moorland model – a small, electric version of a quad bike with chunky tyres, designed for adventurous pensioners. It's not a quad bike, let's get that clear; it is a mobility scooter, just jazzed up for an outdoor existence.

Turns out the scooter lady is a guest of two of the other walkers, who in turn are my family's neighbours. On my GPS tracker, we're a mile and a half from their home. So, they've trekked on foot into a biting headwind. And, despite all of them being at least ten years older than me, they are heading back and so have already traversed the hill on which I've come to a spluttering halt.

This hill is steep and very twisty and going up is a battle, not least because of the loose grit and pebbles washed onto the road, making traction awkward. Going down is somehow worse. Should the lady's scooter skid or the brakes fail she'd fire off into a canyon! Like my mate Eddie 'The Eagle' leaping off a ski jump. Should the worst happen and she disappears over a precipice, we could call her Elderly Edwards. Or Elderly Eagle. To be honest she has more gumption than me, proving once again that I have a cowardly streak.

All four of them stop for a chat and I'm forced to pretend that I'm taking in the scenery rather than on an enforced break. Then we realize that 'Elderly' has vanished. We can see her making stately progress at the bottom of the hill, so my new friends bid me farewell, wish me luck (alarmingly), and leave me to my recovery.

My bike has a natty feature. It's a heavy machine, so to help me push it up steep bits there's a 'walk' button. If I press and hold the headlight button, the bike goes under its own power at walking pace. This, ignominiously, is how I arrive at the crest of the hill. Good job nobody from *Cyclist Plus Magazine* is watching, else I'd have to bribe them not to publish the photos.

This is where I walked the previous day and I confirm that it's my new favourite spot in the world, despite a bitter wind howling across the fells. The birds demonstrate what proficient flyers they are, dipping and soaring, adjusting their wing area and showing amazing control. The sheep give not a jot. They just continue to work their way serenely across the hills, protected by their natural coats. Their progress is slow, but while I've been admiring the view the sheep have moved on in a group and are now out of sight down a gully. Hour after hour, day after day, they graze the fells.

Actually, there is a peculiarity that I'm at a bit of a loss to explain. When we drive towards sheep on the road in the car, they seem unalarmed. A brief, uninterested look and they skip the ditch and shuffle onto the grass at the side of the road to carry on their forage. But when I approach on my bike they scatter to the four corners as if there's a lethal predator among them. Surely I'm not noisier than a car. Not even when I'm wheezing and muttering.

I had studied our host's Ordinance Survey map the previous evening to determine suitable routes for my cycling. I obviously didn't pay enough attention to the contour lines because I had no idea the hills would be so severe. Must do better. Richard is a highly qualified Mountain Leader, so if I tell him about my navigational shortcomings he'll probably scoff and enroll me on a course for idiotic beginners. I'll tell you more about Richard and his walking expertise in due course. For now, I'll merely reflect that I've scratched the surface of a wonderful world.

23

Mr Slightly Ratty

My next ride saw me head north towards the village of Ravenstonedale, about a mile from base. A few hundred yards shy of my destination I encounter Mr Slightly Ratty. He is a less irritable relative of Mr Angry. To start with he had a tooth missing, as do I. However, his is front and centre and obvious. Mine is tucked away at the back where I can store peanuts.

He is the kind of guy who is prepared to talk to a stranger and exchange stories. In fact, as I approach he makes the suggestion of a move into the road, as if to invite me to stop and initiate a conversation. My tales are usually lighthearted, as they are today. He smiles politely at my recollection of Elderly Edwards on her quad-scooter before starting a yarn of his own. His stories start off alright, but they soon degenerate into a bit of a rant against something or other.

For example, he speaks of the fells and local towns and villages with passion. He is a keen walker himself, pointing out distant hills he has conquered. However, before long he ends up spitting and frothing about second-home owners wrecking communities (with some justification, I must add).

His conversation imitates the terrain, switching between gentle rambles and savage hikes. It's like he climbs a hill, gathering frustration as he goes. At the summit, he looks over the edge, a pressure cooker at full steam, eyes wide in a manic, unfocussed stare. He launches himself down the slope. Building up speed, he wails with increasing fervour, a madman on the very limit of control. Reaching the run-off area at the bottom, the storm abates and he is once again a man walking his dog in a bright green valley full of sheep. But he's eyeing the next fell. He's like a knight of yesteryear atop his charger, in full armour, lance at the ready, psyched up, ready for murder. Then along comes old porky on his electric bicycle and Ratty the Knight begins his charge ... (charge, huh? I just realized what I did there).

In my verbal joust with this rampaging horseman, my best weapon is my silky tongue (scant defence indeed). I try and mollify him by changing the subject. He speaks with a pronounced Essex accent, so I ask him how a southerner has ended up in deepest Cumbria.

'Southerner?!' he spits. 'I'm born and bred Cumbrian, as were my parents and grandparents. There's few more Cumbrian than my family.' He explains in his Billericay accent that he went south to make some money. However, he retired at forty-six after the doctor told him that his job as a salesman, with all the inherent hassle of inner London as a territory, would kill him sooner rather than later. So, like me, he wound down commercial activities to the point where neither of us can afford to get our teeth fixed. So, instead of dying in a car smash on the M25 after a heart attack, he returned to his roots with a southern accent which he can't shift. He's been back up north at least ten years, so the change of location has worked. If he could just control his mood swings, he might lower his blood pressure a bit and live to assault yet more fells.

I tell him that some of my family had moved into the area. Not second homeowners, I stress, but full-time living and working folk. He doesn't look too impressed with that so I change tack and say that the lambs are beautiful. I'd taken photos, close up, of beasts that could only be a day or so old. 'Aren't they just the cutest things?' I suggest, showing him a photo on my phone.

'Bloody vegetarians,' he mutters. 'They're everywhere these days. They'll be the death of sheep farmers.'

That is an oblique response to a cheery subject. Time to go before he finds out I don't eat carbohydrates. Conversationally, we never know where that might lead. So, we part company - Mr Slightly Ratty in a vegetarian-induced seethe, me with a smile on my face because I'm in an idyllic corner of England.

* * *

One feature of the area is the light-coloured dry stone walling that defines the fields. I think the walls hereabout are a type of limestone. I did ask Mr Slightly Ratty, but he obviously didn't know because he avoided the question by firing off on an ill-tempered tangent. It's worth knowing what type of stone I might collide with should I be driven off the road by a tractor, so I investigate. Richard has given me some scientific notes on local geology. It's very nearly as complicated as the instructions for the greenhouse I recently constructed.

I discover that limestone is certainly one of the stones used in walling in Cumbria. However, the geology of the area is complex and numerous different types of stone are used, which also require different building techniques. In fact, if I've grasped this to any extent, in (very) general terms there is volcanic rock to the west (the Lake District), largely limestone to the east (the Yorkshire Dales) while here in the Howgills it's mainly sandstone and gritstone. What we have today has developed over the previous 500 million years through the shifting of continents, volcanic activity and, latterly, ice-age glaciation. Right, that's the geological ignorance laid bare - back to the stuff I understand ...

When the morning sun shines, the contrast between the rich, spring grass and the white walls is quite breathtaking. There's a purity about it. One advantage of a bike is that I can see over the walls. Just out of the village, in a field among the ewes and their lambs, I see a hare standing close to a curlew. Before I can disentangle myself and get the phone's camera organised, the hare and the curlew are far away (*The Hare and the Curlew* - could be a poem there). By the time my camera is ready they're somewhere near Windermere, thirty miles distant, one on foot and the other by air. So as not to cause offence to the sheep, who are looking a bit bemused, I reel off a few snaps. Mother sheep looks at my helmeted bonce peering over a wall and decides to lead her young up the hill out of harm's way. I have some way to go to be accepted here.

There are few houses outside the villages, most of them working farms. But there are also plenty of stone-built barns and shelters awaiting a brown envelope in the appropriate planning officer's pocket. Please don't let this wonderful countryside be swamped with new housing. From an initial impression, I'd love to live here, but I would hate the landscape to be spoiled by the likes of me. A rural dichotomy indeed.

24

Tarn Right

One thing about being out in the sticks is that you focus on nature. You notice things because there are so few man-made fripperies to spoil things. Here in the open we are impostors in a worldly production mankind could never create. Out here, the magic of nature is all there is. Apart from a fat bloke with his bike or dog.

Turn right, through a gate, and walk up and over a small hillock and we come across Paradise Tarn. Today is not a cycle day, at least pre-sunrise. It's -4 and my exposed extremities are too vulnerable. So, I walk with the hound. For an hour or more, it will be our own private world. But look closely and there is activity aplenty.

White mist is rolling off a distant hilltop and down a valley. As I crest a rise a pair of hares are startled and dash off across the frosty field. One thing is for sure, it's mighty cold. Yesterday's south-easterly has become a nor'easter and strengthened. It's a blast from the fjords and it really is very cold. We need the sun to work its magic, but that's a good half hour away; even then, progress will be slow. I'm dressed in multiple layers of clothing. Dressed to the 12s in fact; 9s aren't enough.

Below is the tarn. A hundred yards across, perhaps, where a pair of swans and a few Canada geese trawl the lake in splendid isolation. The dog dashes after a rabbit. No chance there. For the dog, that is. There are no sheep in the field surrounding the tarn, so it's safe for the dog to run. We are acutely aware of the vulnerability of the lambs and the farmers' livelihoods. It's hard enough up here without people like me interfering.

This tarn (or corrie) is shallow and it's hard to imagine a large glacier forming here. In fact, it didn't! I just presumed that because it was called a tarn that it really was where a glacier formed. But no, tarn in this instance is being used as a generic term for a Lakeland lake. Tarn may be derived from the old Norse word *tjörn* meaning 'pond.' But Paradise Pond doesn't have quite the same ring to it, so tarn it is.

Here at Paradise Tarn, the land is raised somewhat on three sides, highest at the back, so the basic, classic shape of a glacier is evident, but further investigation reveals that this little lake had nothing to do with glaciation. It's basically a large boggy puddle, though a very attractive one in a stunning setting.

But let's digress a moment because I find glacial tarns interesting. Snow collects in a hollow and compacts to ice. The whole lot rotates backwards and ice 'flows' out at the front. Imagine sliding down a chair and slipping out feet first. What's left when the ice melts is a lake, sealed at the front by the moraine eroded, then deposited, by the glacier. Move on ten thousand years and we have a sanctuary for the birds and a place for the dog and me to frolic. Not frolic perhaps (today it's too cold) – shuffle. In fact, today feels like classic glacier-forming weather.

As the sun creeps up, wildlife cranks into action. Four geese circle us three times before landing on the water. It's a magical sight as they fly before a young sun. Perhaps they're working up an appetite for breakfast. Later in the day, the wind has dropped and it's warmed up so the bike and I are reacquainted. We set off on a mystery tour. I pass the spot, marked by scorched earth, where Mr Slightly Ratty had his meltdown and I find myself beside a lovely old stone bridge over a beck. Up from the beck's bank, over a wall, stand a pair of houses. Typical Cumbrian, solid, rugged, light-coloured stone. Same stone as the bridge and the wall and the scree in the beck. There's a cleanliness about it all; any blemish is likely to be lichen rather than the sooty smears typical of my home town. Nothing really wrong with sooty smears, mind; they are evidence of lives lived and hard graft (and, shamefully, slave-like working conditions at times). The unsullied stone hereabouts has not been interfered with by us, so it's unspoiled. If it wasn't so knobbly, in the words of my Granny, 'it's so clean you could eat your dinner off it.'

Walking towards me along the bank is a man. Not a local, as there was no purpose to his stride. Rather like me, he was just pottering, a guy taking it all in.

'Been coming twelve years,' he says, after I've interrupted his solitude. 'We love it.'

I'm grunting a bit because I'm trying to open the little zip-up bag on my crossbar but my stomach's getting in the way. Oh, the difficulties of a fuller figure. He watches me with some amusement, then tells me he stays in the same holiday house each time he comes, a bungalow in the village. From South Manchester, he comes for the peace and quiet. And there's plenty of that. He didn't seem concerned that a green blob on a bike was sharing his enthusiasm for the area. He could have reacted to me with disdain. Me being an elite athlete after all, dressed for a major cycling tour, utterly out of place in the rugged splendour of Cumbria. But no, he was a simple man able to ignore the bling and seek out the beauty around. It's good to share positive things with a nice man. I like to think that, underneath the flobber and greenery, I'm an ordinary chap too.

His wife had suffered a stroke a couple of years ago and is rather immobile, though thankfully improving slowly. Fortunately, their local accommodation was suitable for her difficulties and they could continue coming to the same place. He told me wistfully that they had managed a short walk together yesterday, but today he was out on his own. There was a sub-text here, namely that he would have loved to have been walking with his wife. He looked up at the distant fells and I could see he wished for fitter, younger days.

Then a quad bike rumbled slowly past, towing a small trailer which contained sacks of animal feed. It was followed by a tractor with a round of hay on a spike on the front. Rush hour in Ravenstonedale. My new friend and I bid farewell and we returned to our own peaceful paths.

25

Quacking Eggs

My machine and I rumble into Ravenstonedale looking like a part-abandoned engineering project. So, what do we discover? It's a very small village to start with. But don't be misled. Don't think the world of enterprise and commerce has passed Ravenstonedale by on the Tebay / Brough road, a couple of hundred yards to the west. Oh, no. Look closely and there's industry aplenty. On a wall in front of a rather splendid house is a plastic Tupperware box. The box is anchored down by an attractive local rock. Next to the box, a sign: *'Duck eggs. Free and tasty. Help yourself.'* (I wonder if the sign advertising duck eggs can be described as a billboard?) I gratefully grab a couple of eggs and wrap them in the spare socks in my rucksack. My local shopping is done for the day.

To get an overview of the place, I cycle boundary to boundary, straight through the village. Even at my speed that doesn't take long. I pass two pubs, both of which have spruced-up outdoor areas to welcome their first customers since the crippling lockdown. There are no shops but there is a defunct junior school (now a children's day nursery), two churches, a number of expensive vehicles, a number of knackered vehicles and a children's play area attached to a tennis court. I wonder whether the posh vehicles belong mainly to urban visitors and the wrecks to local serfs.

There's a beck flowing past the bottom of the village. It's peaceful and gentle now, but I have seen photos of it in flood and it's a different beast.

Just above the beck on the bank are a couple of yurts. These round tents, the approximate shape of a squashed fez, originate on the steppes of Central Asia. One can imagine Attila the Hun having ransacked Kirkby Stephen, four miles north, now resting up in a yurt before his march to lay siege to Kendal. The yurts are pitched not a couple of feet above the beck, so surely they are at risk in times of flood? The catchment areas for all the local waterways are vast tracts of hillside so it's hardly surprising there are floods every now and then. Just had a thought ... perhaps the landowner actually requested a couple of yachts but was misheard.

The larger of the two churches is old, as many tend to be. It's attractive in a simple way and sits squat in the valley, planted on sturdy foundations, permanently hunkered down in expectation of wild winter weather. Evergreen yew trees stand sentinel over ancient graves while their deciduous cousins around the periphery show a hint of spring green, and the grass is tidy. I read that the church is constructed of rubble stone with rusticated quoins. Baffling language indeed for an architectural dunce, so I'm intrigued enough to investigate.

In this most isolated of villages I can research on my telephone; that in itself never ceases to amaze me. I'm sure that modern technology would have made Attila's life easier. Rubble stone is random stuff dug up and used as is, undressed - much like dry stone walls that are built from local stone redeemed when clearing fields for pasture. Quoins are the large cuboid blocks that form the corners of the building. Rusticated means rough. So, there we are - rusticated quoins are rough corner stones. I've learned something. I cycle off feeling smug.

Churches get my attention when I'm idling. Here in Ravenstonedale it's parky, so I need to keep cycling to keep warm. I don't linger too long but it's interesting to look. When we were in France during the summer, temperatures approached forty degrees on occasion, so I'd go into religious buildings to cool off. I wasn't choosy; I would visit small local churches or giant basilicas. To prove I wasn't a mere malingerer, I would study acre upon acre of stained glass window, loitering long enough for my core temperature to drop. I imagine the continental summers in central France could be equally uncomfortable as a nasty Cumbrian winter.

So, what did the locals think of me in their midst? Well, I never found out, because on this particular morning I didn't see another soul. The only evidence of life was the duck egg display. Actually, there were two people. They were playing tennis on the public court across the beck next to the empty kiddies' play area. They were both so well wrapped up, in clothing and their game, that they didn't notice the green blob glide by. Or if they did, they ignored me.

Through town I go off at a tangent down a road that has no signpost at its beginning. It's a road to somewhere and for somebody an actual destination is probably important, but for my meandering it's merely a road to another memory or two. I pass honesty boxes near farms that are doing sidelines. Goat's milk soap is one, various chutneys another. Chutney OK, but I can't help thinking that goat's milk soap is a product of some out-of-dale, arty television programme.

I ride between walls behind which bright green fields are cropped to a carpet by the sheep. Some of the lanes are so narrow that I really don't fancy meeting another vehicle, particularly a tractor, some of which are enormous, towing something that could be even more enormous. I'd have to scramble over a wall or turn round and sprint away. The sprint aspect of my escape plan could prove problematic.

Thankfully vehicles are (unlike me) thin on the ground. The roads are usually around five feet below the wall tops. I can just about see over while riding. I like to stop and stand on the narrow verge between wall and road. This is when it's truly quiet. There is where I hear morning music, a score written on a silent page. The longer I linger, the more it crescendos. The bleating of a lamb, the lower-pitch response by mum. Curlews, carrion-hunting crows, songbirds and geese. There's not a single aeroplane in the blue sky. Somewhere far off I can hear the rumble of a quad bike. These are the modern workhorses of the hill farmer, go-anywhere beasts that tend the sheep, take them extra food or help a struggling lamb. In turn, these lovely animals are the currency of the fells. I utterly respect that and the tough lifestyle that folk hereabouts live.

When the mornings are like this, pristine, I'm reluctant to break the spell. But I must - it's chilly so my feet are suffering. Besides, I've got duck eggs on toast to look forward to.

26

Rural Restoration

When I look up while walking in the fells, I see many things, including kestrels, buzzards, peregrines, songbirds, red squirrels and magical skylines below huge skies. When I look up while walking back home, I'm likely to tread in something unpleasant. I wonder if this is why people walk head down in the urban world. They stare at the ground and examine the way ahead, looking for potholes or avoiding the cracks. Perhaps those that bury themselves in a mobile gadget with a forward camera are actually viewing the pavement on their screens. With eyes or camera, yes, you can dodge a dog dollop, but you don't half miss some interesting stuff above the horizontal. Like sunrises, trees, birds and flowers.

Of course, there are 'country things' lying around up here in the hills too, just not as densely populated. In the bulrushes I come across the sun-bleached, pristine white skeleton of a sheep, picked absolutely clean by native wildlife who've enjoyed an easy meal. A little way away I find the skull. It's peering up at me from deep within the long grass, slowly, slowly dissolving into the earth. This is nature's ultimate recycling.

Close by, there's a small cairn of stones atop a low mound. Someone's pet perhaps, or an old navigation aid. It's nothing too significant; it's barely two feet tall and not on the highest point in the area, but it must have been important to someone. Dotted around the hills and valleys are small stands of trees, including conifers. Isolated islands in the landscape, sometimes with as few as fifteen trees. There are small woodlands of hawthorn, ash and elder, plus I see recently planted beech. But it's the conifers that stand out. Are they planted as a weather-shield perhaps, animal shelters? Sycamores protect isolated farmsteads while also blending in with the landscape, but the conifers look alien. The majority of conifers are evergreens, so perhaps offer shelter all year round? Just out of interest, the word *conifer* literally means 'cone-bearer.' Anyhow, whether groves are natural or man-made, there's plenty of diversity.

There has been a widespread tree-planting programme; thousands of trees all part of a rewilding policy. Outside the areas of managed tree plantations, the landscape is largely bare. It's a huge expanse that appears, at first glance, to be just grassland with the occasional building and odd stand of trees, but there's a lot more to it. It's known as acidic grassland, which sounds noxious but it's not - it's beautiful, and the sheep thrive on it. Many slopes are boggy and known as 'blanket bog,' which attracts ferns and different birds.

I love seeing the sheep slowly easing their way over the moors. I love the lambs in spring and watch them develop over the months and the change each time I visit. I love the wildlife because, as an outsider, it's all new and exciting to me. I find it fascinating that the young sheep are 'hefted,' in other words taught to navigate the fells by their mothers. As most of us live busy urban lives, this magic unfolds unseen to the majority. The teaching and learning goes on generation by generation.

But below the surface and unbeknownst to most people, things are changing. This is evident in those newly planted trees, hundreds of acres of them, many thousands in fenced enclosures. All are native species and include willow, hawthorn, rowan and birch. They are the visible tip of a rewilding programme. It is the cause of much discussion among the people who live, work and visit the area. I like seeing a few sheep dotted about the landscape but I'm beginning to understand that they are not the best use of land, either commercially or environmentally, and there are nowhere near the number there used to be. The harsh reality is that I like this area just as it is. But there is a shift coming, and it's just tough luck on me. People naturally don't like change, but here it appears to be finding favour.

There are grazing rights for 13,500 sheep on the Howgill Fells but only 5,000 sheep actually roam. There's not enough money in it and without subsidies the farmers couldn't survive. So, managing tree plantations is an alternative incentivised income stream. Twenty-four farmers have commoning rights on the Howgills and sheep grazing has dominated fell farming over the last century, but it has resulted in a loss of diversity. That just sounds like one of those soundbites that, to be honest, are spouted by left-wing environmentalists and luvvies. Frankly, most of the time I don't trust these warblings and I think it's the same for other people too - it just goes over our heads. I'm sick of the doom-mongers, and when I stand and look out over this fabulous landscape I don't want anyone telling me it's compromised. In fact, if I'd heard about it while sitting in my armchair in suburbia I wouldn't give it a second thought, but because I'm here and I'm aware that the locals are onside with the changes then I have to pay attention.

I didn't realize that the fells and uplands, as they appear now, are not natural. Heather and wildflowers, for example, have diminished, as have the trees. But things are reverting again. Farmers are being paid to manage wildflower meadows or these new plantations at the expense of sheep. Inside the sheep-free enclosures an increase in scrub, hawthorn and tussocky grass provide foraging and shelter for birds and red squirrels. This boosts the vole population, which in turn stocks the larder for short-eared and tawny owls. Yes, overall, the consequence is that indigenous flora is returning, and with it the wildlife.

In the future, sheep may well be used as a tool to help manage the rewilding. Meat, previously abundant, will become niche, and a premium (expensive) product. As far as I can gather, farmers generally agree with this shift. Previous generations have not made much of a living out of sheep farming, certainly not without the help of subsidies.

The rewilding may actually be described as *unmanaging* the land, in effect allowing it to look after itself with minimal help. It's a large-scale restoration of natural processes which will take decades to take a grip. Today I marvel at the diversity of the area, including the sheep, but if I'm spared for a year or ten, according to environmental forecasters it can only get better. Perhaps I may get to see this lovely area return to what it once was; certainly my younger family will.

It's interesting - the huge landscape is managed now in slow motion by farmers and landowners. What prompted the initial change? Was it the need to feed, or profit and greed? The former, I hope. I know people have to make a living but did the original custodians of the landscape 'rape the land' (in the words of the band *The Eagles*)? I'm trying to imagine the landscape with no 'help' at all, just wild, and I'm struggling. What this man-managed rewilding programme is doing is basically offering just that - 'no help' - but in a managed way, if you get my meaning.

There are patches of heather; in fact towards Kirkby Stephen, on the Sedbergh road, there is a classic heathery moor where I see grouse. I cycle out there one Sunday morning, fairly early, about half-six. Despite the fact that it's an 'A' road, I see only one small van in half an hour, and he stops to check I am OK. I'm actually just putting a bit more air in my tyres, but it was nice of him to stop and ask. Perhaps the cairn I saw earlier was in memory of a lost cyclist! What the lack of traffic does, of course, is to allow the wildlife to go about their business undisturbed, except by the rattling blob on his bat bike.

I spot two more birds which I try (unsuccessfully) to photograph. Instead, I commit them to my prodigious (ahem) memory but fail to find anything similar in the bird book later. Truth is, I couldn't really remember what they looked like when I got back. Further sightings confirm they are probably a whinchat and a ruff, both new to me. Or are they new? What are the chances I've seen them before and not realized? Or not taken the time to have any interest? Whichever, I can now tick them off the list of twitched birds. Just the vast majority of other species remain untwitched. A bird book is generally not something we refer to in the course of our daily lives; most of us are too busy watching TV or clicking our mobile gadget. More's the pity – or rather, moor's the pity.

Every day the stand-out king and queen of birdsong is the curlew. But despite the fact that its song is prevalent, if I tune them out I do hear many others. The lapwing (or peewit) is another wonderful songsmith, but it's in flight where the lapwing wins. Characterised by its broad, rounded wings it performs stunning low-level displays before it rises up, dives again, then zigzags. Amazing aerial skills accompanied by a variety of high-pitch calls.

Whenever I top a crest I can literally see for miles, and invariably there's not a single other person in sight. The wildlife doesn't know how lucky it is to live in such a wonderful place. And they simply don't care about the majority of us living in our fabricated worlds with contrived dreams.

This is the land where wolves once roamed (or was it West Bromwich Albion?). Not sure why I'm thinking about a beast that all but disappeared from England half a millennium ago. Perhaps it's because I can't bear the thought of losing what is before me now. Having said that, if wolves did still roam the landscape and its inhabitants may well be completely different.

A few days ago I was riding up a single-track lane cut into the hillside when I came across a mini-landslip, around ten yards long and eight feet high. Earth and stones had tumbled down to the side of the track. At the point where the slip broke away I saw a miniature snapshot of how a landscape evolves. Just above the slip, at eye level, was a fringe of moorland grass and below that rubbly, sandy soil. Though the slip was obviously recent, there is evidence of new plant life. Below the grassy fringe, tiny ferns are growing – a species of plant that has basically remained unchanged for a hundred million years. And here they are, perpetuating their future as chance allows.

As I've said above, things in the fells are changing. I feel that I've scratched the top layer off and the new reality is just beginning to poke through. I think of those infant ferns growing, remote, at the top of that little landslip a few miles away, and in those bright green shoots see the embryo of widespread change.

I've not seen one black lamb among hundreds, isn't that strange?

One other wonderful sight is fell ponies. I'm not really an equine fan, to be honest. I once stalled a horse on a road that runs through the New Forest. We were on a guided horse walk and mine just stopped. Whatever I tried to get it going, it just sat there. Traffic piled up in both directions as I nudged and shouted at the stubborn sod. Drivers, initially miffed, laughed at my exertions. When we finally got going again it had deposited a steaming mound of fertilizer on the A31 and I vowed never to set foot on a horse again.

So, when the dog and I are confronted by a pair of fell ponies I am rather nervous. One is piebald (black and white) and the other pure black. They have unruly manes like a rebellious teenager and hairy lower legs, like a teenager's dad. Combined with their silky tails, all this excess hair helps keep out the harsh winter weather. To be honest, the horses look magnificent in this wild, wonderful landscape. They are gutsy, rugged animals, clean, fit and free. Thankfully they pay us little interest as I drag the dog past on his lead. Later I find that one pony, the piebald, is the wrong colour and not officially a fell pony at all. A pure-bred Cumbrian fell pony is not allowed to be white. They were both lovely, anyway. Through my binoculars I saw a number of others but this pair were my favourites. In fact, I saw them regularly in various locations, sometimes close by, sometimes on the slopes of a distant fell. Truly free. Unlike some of us, they weren't playing the race card: 'You're the wrong colour. You're not a real fell pony, so you'll have to go live in Yorkshire.' They were just pals wandering the hills, blissfully ignorant of the things that make human interaction so complicated. (Race card - oh dear!)

27

Uther and Arthur

P endragon Castle is described as a romantic ruin. A similar description was leveled at me after I bought my dear wife some flowers for her birthday. The castle is slowly crumbling into the landscape of the stunning River Eden valley. Neither I nor the castle have been ruins forever; both of us were quite impressive in our heydays. I am in the throes of a first physical rebuild while, over the centuries, the castle has had a number of incarnations. My origins have been pretty much authenticated, the castle's less so....

According to the website *Visit Cumbria*:

> '*Pendragon Castle is reputed to have been founded by Uther Pendragon, father of King Arthur. According to legend, Uther Pendragon and a hundred of his men were killed here when the Saxon invaders poisoned the well. There are also claims that the Romans built at least a temporary fort here, along the road between their forts at Brough and Bainbridge. But (apart from legend and supposition), there is no real evidence that there was any building here before the Normans built their castle in the 12th Century.*'

(Mind you, 'Visit Cumbria' has made some assertions about the Ulverston

Canal which are questionable. I'll tell you about them in due course). But legends are good, not least for tourism. Today Mr Porky Green sets out to visit the castle while testing himself and his machine. It's a hilly neighbourhood, you see, and I need to see if the combination of man and bike can cope. If one half fails, the twain are marooned. The human half is the more likely weak link, but we'll see.

Major roads often follow valley floors or hug hillsides. These larger highways are linked by a series of single track lanes with passing places, which tend to wind their way up and over crests. They are often about nine feet wide, asphalt with grass either side, sometimes bordered by rudimentary ditches. From a distance they look like dark grey ribbons laid on the hills - fabulous cycling territory, apart from the sometimes precipitous slopes. This is where the test comes in. Previously, I've only come across one hill where I've ground to a halt because it was too steep. I took a 'private, no entry' road near to where I live, thinking it would be a quick short cut, but I got my just desserts when I ground to a halt and had to turn round. Served me right.

From home base to Pendragon Castle is about 6 miles but there's a few hundred feet of climbs and descents. Total twelve miles with lots of slopes. Battery and man need to do the whole dozen miles because running out of juice with a mile to go could be a real nuisance. The bike is 25 kilos and shoving it up a steep hill would not be much fun. The first four miles are on wider roads, the last two on twisty, hilly 'ribbons.' There are a number of steep battery-sapping inclines before I get to the highest point, about a mile from the castle. I pause at the top to have a drink (water, in case you're wondering). I've just passed a parked car. It's one I saw two days ago in the same spot. As I look back, it's slightly below me, 30 yards off the road. There's really nothing else up here except sheep and birds and I wonder if all is OK.

In the true public-spirited attitude that has served mankind through the ages I don't bother checking and set off down the hill. It's at least a mile, and some of it pretty steep. The only danger on the way down is driving into a ditch or pile of rocks, which would be pretty stupid and I wouldn't tell you about that if I did. Part way down is a parking spot. In it there's a rather smart estate car, the owner of which is trying to pitch some sort of tent. He waves as

I zoom past. Down and down the twisty road, ever more mindful that I have to come back up. Near the bottom I pass a house that used to be a farm - not the first such arrangement. Lots of farms and attendant buildings are now homes to non-farming incomers, living in rural isolation outside native lore.

My narrow ribbon is called Tommy Road and the castle is at the junction of it and the 'B' road which connects Kirkby Stephen to all points south, including Hawes, and Wensleydale cheese. I'll tell you about that later too! The bigger road I've joined is one of those with an unmissable blue sign at its start: '25 *motorcyclists have been seriously injured on this road in the last 2 years.'* Pretty cheerful welcome, I think you'll agree.

The castle is a ruin - it won't be keeping Uther or Arthur dry without a new roof, at the very least. But it's absolutely charming and deserted. It's in a private field, a grazing habitat, and as such is closed off by a strongly-sprung five-bar gate.

I'm not only worried about my battery running out, I'm also bothered about having the bike pinched because it was pretty expensive. Plus, I don't want to walk back. So I decide to take it through the gate and hide it behind the wall, away from thieving eyes, while I explore. Actually, it doesn't go quite as smoothly as that. The bike is quite weighty and the spring on the gate is very strong. The gateway itself is rutted from tractors going in and out (and dragons?). At this point I'm glad there's nobody else about because I make a complete mess of the following three minutes.

I have to wheel my bike through while holding the gate open against the strong spring. Halfway through, my wheels get caught in a deep tractor rut and there follows a slow motion shambles. I fall over and end up in the mud, trapped underneath my bike. Then the gate creaks closed on its heavy spring, in turn trapping both me and the bike. I'm lying on my back like a corpulent green beetle stuck under a scrap heap. If someone had choreographed this as some sort of comedic stunt, it wouldn't have worked. 'Too contrived ... utterly unrealistic', they would cry. 'Nobody could possibly make such a balls-up of going through a gate.' Took me a while to extricate myself, I can tell you. I bet Uther didn't have this trouble, but at least I gave his ghost a giggle.

The castle is charming. Indeed, as wrecks go, it's a good one (can you tell

I'm being a bit peevish because of my battle with the gate?) From an overhead photo you can see a grass moat around the castle. Local legend says that Uther tried, unsuccessfully, to alter the course of the nearby River Eden to fill the moat, giving rise to the well-known couplet (locally anyway):

Let Uther Pendragon do what he can,
Eden will run where Eden ran.

Drifting through this lovely landscape is a whiff of legend-based commercialism. Just across the road from Pendragon Castle is Pendragon View. Without the legend that is King Arthur it would be 'Pile of Stones View.' I'm half expecting to see Pendragon's Ice-creams drive up or Uther's Kebabs. Much more of this and we'll have a Loch Ness Monster situation – a contrived drip feed of nonsense that's kept tourists coming to Scotland for about ninety years. It's a good job Nessie is long-lived or a whole industry would be furloughed. Of course, now they can add 'Fatso's Gate' to the marketing blurb - that'll bring 'em flocking. On a return visit at a later date, I spot something previously unnoticed - a post box. There are perhaps two houses within a mile and no town for about three, so what on earth a post box is doing out here is a mystery. I can only assume it is part of Uther's marketing plan: 'Pendragon's Post Box - campaign donations here, please.'

The castle is open to the elements and looks rather rickety. I believe that visitors can clamber where they will; there are no restrictions. Actually, this is not true. I've missed a perfectly good warning notice posted on the gate expressly forbidding people to walk on or within the ruins - something I did with the unbounded enthusiasm of a beetle scurrying over a sheep dropping. I probably missed the sign because I was lying underneath the gate on which the sign had been nailed.

Anyhow, as I cavort around the mossy stones, a foot wrong here or a slip there could result in injury. I presume that the Health and Safety guidelines were put together by Uther, back in the days when his subjects were expendable. If you're lying injured you can take your mind off things by marvelling at the lovely small blue flowers growing from the cracks in the walls, nature's nod of sympathy to the people who lived a brutal existence in the castle. The flowers are possibly campanula, though I'm not well up on ancient flora.

From the ramparts there are stunning views over the River Eden valley and up the towering fells. It is a magical place. I can imagine standards flying from the towers as horses clip-clop along the valley floor, returning home from massacring somebody. Various rooms are evident, though it's not clear what was what. Though, if I have my ancient architecture right, I think I recognize the 'bathroom' with its outlet, like a chimney stack, down the outside wall. The exterior walls are thick and solid and, though the structure looks quite small from a distance, it's evident that constructing it would have been tough work. Close up, it's pretty imposing. I think maybe it looks small because of the vast landscape it's set in.

Not sure why, but as I look out over the river my mate John comes into my thoughts. The river would have been a means of defence and a source of nourishment. I think specifically of the 'Responsibly Sourced Fish' slogan that you see on packets these days. Well, it doesn't come any more responsible than my mate because he never catches anything. I can see him sitting on the canal bank, laughing and enjoying the scenery. I'm sharing a pleasant day with an absent friend. Think I might need a psychotherapist?

Time to go. I prop the gate open with a big log, then take my bike out. I'm not getting stuck again. Learning on the job, you see. The battery monitor shows plenty of charge as I begin my ascent. It does look quite a long way up as the road disappears over a distant crest. It will look a very long way if have a 'mechanical incident' but I'm soon buzzing uphill quite nicely. Don't think I'm doing no work; the bike is not self-driven - it needs rider input. 'Electrically assisted' is the term. I have to put effort in, especially on the very steep bits, so about two-thirds of the way up I'm ready for a breather . The man with the posh car has had a rethink and taken his tent across the road to a flat bit of grass, presumably where there's more room to manipulate poles and canvas. I ask politely if he's staying in his tent overnight.

'It's a shelter,' he tells me curtly, 'not a tent.'

I sense that things are not progressing as anticipated. Then suddenly from nowhere, a wicked little gust of wind whips in and the canvas flips up in the air like a discarded paper bag. While trying to hang on to prevent it disappearing over the fells, he releases his hold of the poles - which collapse in a heap with a clang. As I leave he's underneath the canvas cursing his wife who is, 'not helping at all, dear.' I set off again chortling, which is not ideal for big uphill breaths. But Columbanus does me proud and we reach the top. Two bars out of four showing on the battery monitor, all good so far. Five miles to go and the very steepest of the climbs done with.

The car that I gallantly ignored on my way in is still there. Car number two (of two) in this enormous landscape. No sign of life. A little guilty at my previous disregard for someone in potential trouble, I decide I'd better take a peek and ride over the sheep-cropped grass to investigate. I tentatively peer in. There's a chap lying in the car on a sleeping bag. His head is in the boot with his feet on the flattened passenger seat. He looks very comfy actually, but he's worryingly still. Exactly what he thought of my ruddy, blue-helmeted face pressed up against his window when he opened his eyes I'm not sure, but he certainly gave me quite a start when he sat up. He was staring at me with a mixture of fury, terror and panic. He wound the window down.

'Sorry,' I said, 'I was just making sure you are OK.'

'Right,' he replied, blinking wildly. 'Thank you. But if I'd been dead it wouldn't have mattered, would it?' He raised his eyebrows. I had to concede he had a point.

'Actually,' he continued, 'I've just got back from the pub where I had a couple of pints and a big meal. That was preceded by a long walk. Consequently, I was taking an afternoon nap.'

'Oh,' I said. 'That's alright then.'

After he'd had a monster yawn, we actually had quite a decent conversation. Nice chap he was, from Newcastle, who had been to the same spot a few times before. One of his favourites he told me, and I could see why. I told him that now I knew his habits, I wouldn't disturb him in future.

'Very considerate,' he mumbled.

I decided that this was my equal favourite Cumbrian spot, alongside the one where I saw the lady on the scooter. I suspect I may find other equal favourite spots. It's the top-of-the-worldness of it, the silence, the vast skies and the uninterrupted views, at least till the next range of hills, which can be ten or twenty miles distant. Around me, just the birdsong and (if there's no wind) the gentle sound of the sheep chomping on the grass, a man battling with a misbehaving tent and another trying to get a bit of kip.

The bike does me proud and we get home with a bit of charge left. That's been a great ride.

28

Ghost Town

To get my creative juices going I cycle and walk. Not sure whether the cobwebs get blown out or inspiration gets blown in. Sometimes I do concentrate and take in my surroundings, but other times I wander around in neutral. Let's be honest, more often than not I'm in neutral. I sometimes just set off without any sort of plan and see what happens.

For example, while on a mystery tour bike ride yesterday I found myself at a little crossroads. There's a sign to a place called Barras, which sounded interesting - 3 miles. I've got the satnav on my phone to make sure I'm not too far from home if the battery gets low. I ride along a delightful lane between alternate walls and hedgerows, birds singing, sheep bleating. I've gone two and a half miles when I get to a 'T' Junction. Right to Barras, two and a half miles! Either I'd missed a turn somewhere, which I didn't think was the case, or there was a signpost / distance-measuring issue.

I never do find Barras. It appears to be a place of myth. I research and find that it used to have a railway station and used to be in Westmorland. I think Westmorland is a nice-sounding place for a village to find itself. Unfortunately, Westmorland was de-frocked (or whatever happens to out-of-favour counties) and incorporated into Cumbria, so now Barras is a place that nobody can find in Cumbria. I do find twenty 'things of interest to do in or near Barras,' but I can't find Barras itself. As I cycle in circles I half expect to find Hogwarts round the next bend of the non-existent railway line in a defunct county. All rather mysterious. If anyone actually lives in Barras, would you be so kind as to drop me an email?

On the way back I stop atop a knoll. It's sunny, clear and nothing stirs; it really is pretty isolated. Then, on the ground, I spot a used tea bag and a 20p piece. I leave the tea bag where it is (biodegradable) and set off again - slightly annoyed that whoever it was didn't leave more cash. I continue on my ribbon, aiming to reach a waterfall I have previously seen in the distance from my favourite spot. It's hidden from view up a small valley. I leave the bike (locked up, though there's probably no need) and stride out, but slowly. This is an isolated spot. Once round a bend I'm out of sight of the road and there's no knowing when somebody will actually pass this way. My legs are a bit fragile so I'm wary of busting one. Being in a small valley within a fold in the fells there's no phone signal, so I'm unsure if an emergency call would get through. The terrain underfoot is alternately boggy and rocky as I'm walking beside an old stream; it has carved out a steep-sided course which is very slopey at times. A missed footing and I could slither into a chilly beck.

Just yesterday, while walking nearby, I came across a memorial stone engraved with the names of a local couple. It was roughly 9 inches by six and completely invisible from any road or path; it was pure fluke that I happened upon it. It is set into a grass bank above a beck. What a wonderful place for a man and wife to be at rest. Their names are engraved black on a white background. From where they lie you look over the beck at the hillside which climbs way up. The only sounds are the chattering brook and a host of birds. Just to finish off it all off, the sheep have neatly trimmed the grass around the plaque.

Today I find a painted stone, I presume done by a child. The stone is about six inches across and worn smooth by the stream from where it's been rescued. Whoever it was has painted a rudimentary picture of a sheep's head and written below, *'Thank you God for Sheep.'* Sheep are all around, have been for many years, and they and their custodians comprise a large part the local way of life - someone is paying homage.

The waterfall is perhaps a quarter of a mile from the track, though it feels more because of the chaotic terrain. En route I pass another sheep's skeleton, once again picked clean. The water up here in the stream is as fresh as it gets, seeping off the fells and channelled into rivulets. I have a well-earned drink and have the unsavoury thought that I've quite likely ingested a decent percentage of sheep's piss. Just another healthy addition to eons-old minerals washed from the soil.

The waterfall is around ten feet high and chatters down over rocks into a fresh, clear pool. I imagine a children's author have her characters visit here as part of a daring childhood adventure where they'll learn about mythical creatures of the fells from the spirits of long-dead beasts who roam the moors.

My little waterfall is piddly compared to the one we saw a couple of days ago - namely Cautley Spout, not far from Sedbergh. The water tumbles about 650 feet down a series of waterfalls. Nearby is the Cross Keys Temperance Inn. Yep, no booze. Apparently, the landlord died while helping a pickled punter home and the new landlady banned the drink thereafter. We're still in lockdown so we couldn't go in, but I read somewhere that if you visit in the evenings you're likely to bump into teachers from nearby Sedbergh School. Must be different to my school because non-drinkers are not the kind of teachers I had!

III

Part Three

Further ramblings from the north and beyond ...

29

So Long, ago

Today we're heading out on a nostalgic pilgrimage. Our destination is a tiny hamlet called Kentmere. It's four miles up a single-track road, heading east off the Kendal / Windermere Road. We're aiming for the Grove Hotel. It was from there that my uncle began his last walk. He was a keen trekker and a regular guest at the hotel, which was run by a lady called Mrs Driscoll. In October 1979 my uncle set off on a major trek across the hills. He confided to Mrs Driscoll that he didn't feel very well. Despite her telling him to stay and rest, he set off. A mile into the walk he collapsed and died of a massive heart attack. It transpires that he had a congenital heart condition but hadn't told anyone.

I was in Canada at the time and it was my mum who wrote with this sad news. She said that he died doing exactly what he wanted. It would have been awful to watch an active man gradually decline and, despite the shock and sadness of his death, it was in all honesty a good way to go and the way that he would have wanted to go. But, far too early, aged just 55.

The road up to Kentmere rises gently all the way. It's narrower than I remember and seems much more than four miles. We're hemmed in all the way by dry stone walls so I have to concentrate. Passing places are few but thankfully, despite roads in general being far busier, we meet only one vehicle all the way up.

My recollections are rather hazy. I have visited the Grove Hotel on a few occasions and stayed at least once, but most recently around four decades ago. The fell rising up behind the hamlet looks steeper and more imposing, and it feels colder than I remember. In fact, I don't recognize the building from the road. The trees are bigger and there are more bushes, so perhaps my memory is playing tricks. It's only when I go through a gate and peer down a short drive that I recognize a single storey extension that used to be the hotel bar.

I'm looking around gormlessly when a man comes out of the door. I'm on his private drive and he looks a bit perturbed, so I explain what I'm up to. When he's assured that I'm neither a Jehovah's Witness nor a marauding vagrant, he tells me that he bought the property in 2002 from Mrs Driscoll herself. She seemed old when I visited, so it's nice to know she remained there for a further twenty plus years. It's good to speak with the gentleman and have a direct link to the times I recall. He tells me that Mrs Driscoll's husband died in 1983, though I have no recollection of him at all. Mrs Driscoll continued on her own but failing health, and anno domini, led to the business gradually winding down. It must have been terribly hard running a hotel on her own in this isolated, end-of-the-line hamlet, though I believe they accommodated the occasional wedding in later years with the help of some ladies in the village.

Just as he's getting to the pith of his explanation my wife rushes up and asks if she can use his loo! Then our car alarm starts going off. 'That'll be the dog bouncing about in the car, furious at being left alone in perfect rabbit-hunting territory,' I explain. Fortunately, our host is a tolerant chap and he carries on with his history lesson. He tells me that there's a lady living just up the hill who has been in the hamlet all her life. She would have directly bridged the year gap for me, but I don't want to alarm anyone else. Considering he bought the place back in 2002, it's still a place in transition, but without doubt it's a wonderful house in a stunning location. Having said that, I wouldn't have recognized it at all if he had demolished the bar! He's concentrated on other areas and I think he has built extensions on the side. Perhaps he left the bar till after my visit. Squaring a circle, if you will, allowing me to put the 1970s to rest. They were, in all truth, a pretty turbulent time for me and our family.

Despite our uninvited intrusion we part company on friendly terms. I bid my new acquaintance thanks and farewell and he goes back through the door my uncle and I would have used all those years ago. I stand in reflective quiet for a few minutes. Forty years on I'm a different person. The house and village look smaller. Perhaps these days the buildings are dwarfed by large trees. The fells all around are more imposing and threatening. That's probably because I'm older and physically less capable. Less like a fearless child on a bike.

My uncle was a gregarious chap, quick with a laugh and the foil for my mother's faux frustration at his eccentricity. They loved each other dearly. I gave him a lift to the train once when he was off on a walking holiday in Austria. Bear in mind that he lived on the twentieth floor of a block of flats in the centre of Rochdale, a place he'd chosen temporarily after his mother died twenty years previously. He was an anesthetist but had never psychologically got over her death, never settled down. I arrived at the flats early in the morning to find him dressed and fully equipped for an alpine climb. 'They'll all be dressed properly when I pick up the boat train in London,' he said.

When he got back he laughed when he told me that even when he got to the tiny station that was his Austrian destination in the Alps, people were still dressed in suit and tie. I can sense his laughter carried away on the breeze as he sets off excitedly on his last adventure. I can hear the crunch of his boots on the gravel as he begins his final climb up Harter Fell. I was 3,000 miles away when he died but today, finally, I've come to wave him off and wish him a safe journey.

Note:

The current owner has generously responded to my request for information relating to the history of the hotel, particularly in the 1970s. He emailed me some photographs, one of which is from (he believes) 1975. It's a wonderful shot, taken from the air. It is so distant in my memory it could have been taken by the Montgolfier brothers! In fact, the shot itself is summer hazy, reflecting my recall. And yes, it certainly does bring back memories. But, going off the photo, even back then the trees look substantial and the place is rather larger than I remember - meaning my memory is skewed. Perhaps the physical memories have been overwhelmed by emotion and time.

These extra notes sent to me by the current owner offer an interesting snapshot of the development of a Cumbrian hamlet over the years:

About half of the houses in Kentmere are built on the foundations of houses dating from 1500 or so. The Grove is such a building. They were all customary tenements of the absentee Lord of the Manor. From the evidence of the several which still retain some of the original timbers, these houses were thatched single-storey buildings. The evidence of thatch is easily seen on the weathered upper surfaces of the 'A' framed roofs and the various mortices show the structural shape precisely. It can be taken that there were all 'farmsteads' in those times. As the population grew and the value of the customary rent (constant 13s-4d, or 67 pence in modern money) became ever of less concern as the result of inflation, then the more prosperous enlarged their properties. In the 17th and 18th centuries they changed them to two-storey buildings. Apart from a few of the older buildings, these would all have been farms and the Grove was such right up to the beginning of the 20th century. Advances in animal husbandry by this time dictated that larger barns were needed and those farms with flat ground appear to have prospered more than others, for obvious reasons.

The Grove on its steep land thus passed out of being a farm in its own right, becoming simply one of several within a larger estate with accommodation let to non-farming labour - even though still with its barn used by the wider estate. The main estate in which it fell came up for sale in the 1950s after 70 years in the same hands (a Penrith gentleman) but this being a very difficult time for hill farming the Grove was sold out of it to the Driscolls in 1956 by executors. The main estate didn't find a buyer until a few years later. The Grove became a tearoom (again, as it had been temporarily in 1949) and then with a sign for 'Morning Coffee, Bar Snacks and Teas' gradually enlarged to B&B status, and finally as a Guest House with H&C running water in bedrooms! ('Hotel,' I think, is too grand a name as it implies live-in staff. There is no account of there being live-in staff, even when it had 7 bedrooms). Mrs D managed to continue after 1983 for a while with help from several Kentmere ladies, but it was never going to last. A few local wedding receptions were held in later years but paying guests became few: it had been such a big part of her life that she didn't want to go, but health dictated that she needed more hospitable accommodation – there are 14 different levels in the house!

30

Grange-over-Grass

.....which used to be Grange-over-Sands. The bay has silted up so there's grass where there used to be beach. It is a sixty-metre-wide strip between the shore and Morecambe Bay. Some of it is stable enough for sheep to forage.

We're making a whistle-stop tour of the towns of southern Cumbria, the major ones anyway, starting with Grange - which to me has always had that classy Victorian away-day image. In fact, I'm wrong; I learn it's Edwardian. We're looking for somewhere to live. We already live in a nice town in a house on which we've put a great deal of effort. But we're always on the lookout for the next adventure. I don't like the idea of a final resting place, it's too permanent, too 'end of the line.' And if we're going to have a change, I've always fancied living by the sea – along with the rest of the world who've realized that living in a city during a pandemic is a poor idea.

Grange is a hilly town suited to tourists with goat-like surefootedness. Residents will likely be (largely) retired people who can cope with changes in altitude. It looks to be a town in transition, with a number of properties undergoing renovation, so scaffolding causes some congestion on the narrow streets. The shops look independent and interesting as opposed to the 'chain' shops one usually sees. Mind you, most of them are closed!

High on its list of attractions is an Ornamental Lake (Duck Pond). It advertises a wide variety of waterfowl, gaily coloured birds which have migrated from distant shores. Sadly, most of the birds have been stolen!

According to the blurb it costs between £40 and £110 each to replace the birds, which is probably why there's more water than bird on view. They've had to cross out 'ornamental' and 'wildlife' so it's now, Grange-over-Grass Pond. Unfortunately, that doesn't have quite the same allure. It's sad because locals have produced an information board and colour leaflets showing how good it used to be. Mind you, the birds that are here today look perfectly happy. They included some bar-headed geese, a new one on me. I read they breed in Central Asia, so they've had quite a trip! Perhaps there aren't many places with enough space where they can just be themselves. The remaining birds are just not attractive enough to the bird rustlers. Bit of an avian confidence-knocker this. Perhaps it's why they look a bit mournful.

The pond, despite being short of wildlife, is very pleasant actually, set in a park full of mature fir trees. The authorities have sited the public loos in the park ensuring a steady stream of visitors (if that's the right expression).

Without doubt Grange is a tourist town, well known and of good repute, but it looks rather weary. The pond felt drained of cheer, which seemed a metaphor for the town itself. I hope it's because we're in the last throws of Covid restrictions and the decline is not terminal. Actually, I think it will be fine. There are always tourists and I'm sure they will come back. According to the scuttlebutt, there are a number of towns around the south of Cumbria that are reputed to have a great future behind them. We'll see. I hope not.

However, there is a splendid promenade here. Not attached to the town, mind you - it's some way south. In fact, you have to be pretty fit to walk to the promenade. But there's plenty of (paid) parking, though not close by any means. There's a café on the prom where I have a sausage. It would have been a sausage sandwich but I'm off bread. To be honest, the lack of bun lays bare the sausage's weakness. Not a gourmet titbit. But I'm served by a very pleasant lass who is delighted that her establishment is open again after a dismal lockdown. She must have one of the nicest working environments anywhere - her café looks straight out over the bay and, on a sunny day like this, it's wonderful.

Sitting at one of the café's tables, sited on the prom, we come across a very nice gentleman with whom we share a pleasant half hour. He's an elderly chap who lives across the bay in Arnside, at the eastern end of the railway viaduct which crosses the bay away to our left. This is his first trip out since the easing of lockdown restrictions and he's tucking into his sandwich and brew with some determination. He takes the train from Arnside, across the viaduct round to Grange station. From there he walks the mile-long promenade with the help of his wheeled walk-aid. He's somewhat restricted physically, but he's doing his best to ignore that. He's a guy who is getting out and enjoying his twilight years in a wonderful spot. He'd probably be enjoying it rather more if I didn't keep pestering him. In this land of rugged terrain and mountains he's done well to find a flat bit. In fact, the only other flat area is Morecambe Bay itself. But best to avoid that - his chariot might get a bit bogged down in there.

Hang on! The chap has told us that he walks the mile from Grange, yet we were signposted to a paid car park well away from the town. If there was access to the prom from the town, we never found it - or were deliberately ushered south!

Whatever misgivings I have about man-made additions, like parking ticket machines, the landscape and vistas hereabouts are truly magnificent. I read that the air was particularly good for Edwardians with tuberculosis, so there's no reason to think that it's not equally good these days. Unless one factors in the murderous potential of Heysham Nuclear Power station 15 miles across the bay. Oh, and Sellafield Nuclear reprocessing plant 40 miles northwest. Then there's Chernobyl. Considering they only lifted restrictions on the final Cumbrian sheep farms in 2012, 26 years after the nuclear plant sent over its noxious cloud, maybe Grange is not a good choice after all. Or if we do end up here, we'll just have to stop eating grass and have an underground bunker on hand.

While sitting outside the café we can see the tide coming in, literally. Over the grass 'beach,' fifty yards away, there's a small wave, or bore, running up the narrow channel on our side of the bay. It looks to be moving at a good walking pace and as the channel fills it isolates the huge sandbanks out in the bay. It all looks rather dangerous. Of course, it's not far from here where tragedy struck. Twenty-three Chinese cockle pickers were stranded by the tide and drowned. They were, I believe, illegal immigrants just trying to make a better life for themselves. The suspicion is they were being exploited for their cheap labour. A truly miserable episode.

But overall, Grange-over-Grass. Tick.

31

There's a lot when you Look

Four days ago I had a typical ride on a bike in and around Ravenstonedale. Starting at 6.07 AM, I cycled sixteen miles - which felt like sixty because of the cruelly cold wind. To make matters worse, most of it was uphill (I don't seem to notice the downhill bits!). Until I consciously think about it, I don't realize just how much is going on around me.

Trundling around the countryside that morning I saw about 200 sheep (some lying in hollows, possibly frozen to the ground), one car, two duck eggs (left in a 'help-yourself' box on a wall, which I did - for the second time!), two curlews (but heard more), a buzzard, a black grouse, two pairs of lapwing, plenty of geese, ducks, swans, a number of red squirrels, countless rabbits, three hares, a rat (on the patio), a mouse (in the kindling basket), a woodpecker, and pied and grey wagtails. I'm going on record here to say that the grey wagtail's name does not do it justice. Sure, there's a bit of grey on it, but it's largely yellow below decks and a lovely colourful bird. In fact, I'm going to write to the ornithological high-ups and moan like mad. I notice non-animal things, too. Derelict barns and shelters, for example, petrified into the landscape by the numbing frost.

At the end of it all (about an hour and a half) there were two tired legs belonging to one very knackered cyclist who treated himself to a pair of duck eggs on toast after a hot shower. Three days later I had recovered sufficiently to write up the experience and continue life.

* * *

We've had sheep in the garden but have no idea how they got in. Everywhere is enclosed by fence or wall. Sure, sheep can jump and scramble over walls and fences, but they are leaving no clue as to where they are breaching our defenses. I have forensically examined the whole perimeter and found no evidence of ovine obtrusion. There's no barrier under about five feet, so if that's how they're getting in they are not only pretty accomplished woolly jumpers but also experts at leaving no spoor to follow. There is a cattle grid on the drive which is a deterrent, certainly for cows at least. But now I learn that sheep in Wales have learned how to cross a cattle grid by rolling over them on their backs! Ovine evolution in the land of the leek. Has word of this cunning means of ingenious ingress spread to Cumbria?

Close-up, sheep are actually engaging creatures who sport a permanent grin and look at you through a slit-pupiled eye. But I have a question. How many sheep do you need to form a flock? Something else my addled brain idled about while loitering. Two? No, I don't think so. Twenty sheep would be considered a flock, so somewhere between two and twenty is the beginnings of a flock. Sheep display flock-like tendencies in a gathering of five (or another source says four, and another still says three!), so perhaps there lies the answer – three, four or five. A 'small' flock in Australia can be thousands, in the USA under a hundred. And, the very term 'flock' can be open to interpretation. It can mean sheep gathered together by a farmer or animals that stay together when not forced to. Confusing, eh?

* * *

Newbiggin-on-Lune straddles the A685 running along the valley floor. The fells rise either side and both directions are memorable on a bike. Head north up onto Orton Fell. Lovely up here on a summer's morning but, boy, I bet winter is bleak. One ribbon road amid miles of open moor. This little road is appropriately named High Lane and within a few hundred yards I'm climbing up into the hills, a world away from the busy main road below. It's literally another world with other-worldly names. Nettle Hill is to my right, Great Asby Scar to my left, ahead Crosby Garret Fell. Little Asby (I really want to put an 'H' in there but there isn't one) is a couple of miles further along. But as I cross Potts Beck immediately before two farms, one either side of the ribbon, my way is blocked by a herd of cows. There are twenty or so untended beasts, wandering along the road between dry stone walls, and I'm reluctant to interrupt their morning ramble. Let's be honest, I'm a bit fearful that I might go down in a hail of bullocks. So I just sit and listen to the waking moors, then turn round and head back up the moor. In the space of a couple of miles I've traversed a fell, a scar, a hill and now a moor (though that's my word for it - it just looks like a moor).

This little snapshot of a few minutes in the hills charges my imagination. I'm in Cumbria but also in the North Yorkshire National Park. It was laid down as such in 1954, three years after Derbyshire's Peak District, which was our first National Park. Although it's a national treasure, 95% of the park is in private ownership. As I (and many thousands of others) visit and appreciate this wonderful landscape it's worth taking a moment to say thank you to the farmers, businesses and property owners who look after the land on our behalf. A lot is down to the sheep who trim the moors and fertilize them, but somebody has to look after the sheep in wintertime or through lean years.

In fact, as we travel through this beautiful area, much of what we see has been laid down by people in times gone by. They created what we see today just by living the lives they did. Flower-filled meadows, hedgerows, patchwork fields within thousands of miles of dry stone walls, centuries-old shelters scattered across the fells built to protect the animals in harsh times.

It's all well and good for the yellow blob to be charging around the moors having fun on a balmy summer's day. But try and imagine farmers tending their animals in what must be brutal conditions as snow is driven unchecked across the moors. They are doing the hard yards in the long, dark months to keep themselves afloat and make sure that they can try and prosper when the warmth returns. And we, the outsiders, benefit.

South from Newbiggin there's a ribbon towards Weasdale. Bessy Beck trout fishery's twin pools are ice-still, apart from the odd ripple as a trout grabs a breakfast insect. It's a wonderful ride through yellow-topped gorse. A simple wooden sign points the way up Green Bell which gently slopes away up the hill, inviting the fit to have a go. I cycle on to Weasdale Nurseries, which looks like it's been abandoned - lockdown again. Mind you, it's still early; no opportunity to mess someone's day up with pithy conversation. This little road is peace personified.

The contrast between where we are here in rural northern England and cycling in cities cannot be starker. On one occasion, we were on the boat, moored in Islington on Regent's Canal in North London. The mooring is in a cutting, above which manic life rushes on. I'd arranged for some post to be delivered to a hotel so had to cycle in to pick it up. It was a couple of miles each way. The date was 9/7/2005. This is two days after the 7/7 London bombings when the underground and a bus were targeted by terrorists.

Cycling through London that day, setting off at 5.45 AM was quite an experience. Even at that hour, there were many police in evidence, a reassuring presence for Londoners trying to maintain a normal routine. One group were guarding the end of a street completely blocked by a white 10-foot-high barricade, behind which they were investigating the site where the bus was bombed. It was a peculiar feeling being so close to the site of an atrocity when my only previous awareness of it was via television. Then, I was safe in my arm chair, distanced, but today I witness the aftermath close to and that is very sobering. At this time of day it is pretty quiet; there is some traffic but you can feel the city waking up, aware that a human tsunami is gathering out to sea ready to crash in and swamp unwary cyclists. By the time I return to the boat at around 7.00 AM, Islington is truly awake. Horns parp and engines roar as people disappear into the underground station like termites into their hill - normal people, brave and determined to cock a snook at those trying to murderously disrupt their lives.

Frankly, I am relieved to disappear back to the canal protected deep in its canyon. I ride on rural towpaths where I compete with the odd dog walker or fisherman. But it's different in and around towns and cities; particularly how the towpaths are increasingly being used as highways for cyclists and joggers - weekday commuters, weekend thrill-seekers. One thing they have in common is their total lack of communication with each other or me. There appears to be an utter lack of awareness of anything going on around them. Eyes down, headphones on, they're in a world of their own. 'Serious' cyclists in Lycra shorts, helmets and wrap-around sunglasses look deadly serious, desperate not to be passed by librarians and secretaries riding sit-up-and-beg 'commuter cycles' - ordinary folk on their way to work and wearing business attire and rectangular horn-rimmed spectacles like the headlights on a sit-on lawnmower.

Everyone is dead serious; they don't appear to be enjoying it in the slightest. A tide of urban angst, removed from the world beyond, wrapped in their own spheres. There seems to be a desperation to get wherever they are going, as if arriving at the source of income is to arrive at a place of safety.

I do like to visit towns and cities, but before most folk wake up. The thing I love about the fells is the space and freedom, not only of movement but also of thought. The backdrop is the call of bird, a place where I can take lungfuls of fresh air and let my imagination go.

32

Canal Foot

Ulverston Canal is the 'shortest, widest, deepest canal' in England, according to Alan Postlethwaite writing on the *Industrial History of Cumbria* website. It's also claimed to be the straightest! It's 1¼ miles long, 15 feet deep and 66 feet wide. For anyone vaguely familiar with canals, the combination of these statistics certainly make it very unusual. However, the Wardle Canal is shorter (154 feet) and the Manchester Ship Canal is deeper (up to 30 feet) and wider (up to 80 feet). And the New Junction Canal in South Yorkshire is as straight as an arrow, too. But let's not let facts get in the way of a fascinating little snippet of waterways history.

For us, the canal is a most unexpected thing to happen upon. We were heading for Ulverston town centre but I missed the sign. To get over that disappointment, I decided to stop for lunch. Bit of a non-sequitur, but there we are. Looking for somewhere to park, I followed a sign for Canal Foot, attracted by the name purely because I'm a canal lover. I'd no idea there was a canal in this area (the nearest being the Lancaster Canal some forty miles distant). I certainly wasn't expecting to find either a canal or a foot. But I found both.

The Ulverston Canal stretches from a basin in the town to Morecambe Bay. It is no longer serviceable, not least because there's a concrete lock gate at the canal exit. The inner lock gate looks original and unmaintained. It's a skeletal steel frame attached to some rotting timber. Historic or authentic, one may (optimistically) describe it. Or knackered. The next time it moves it will be into a skip. There's also a modern road bridge across the centre of the lock - access north for walkers, cyclists and local residents.

Canal Foot sounds like a boating ailment; instead it's a wonderful little oasis. It helps that the weather is perfect. During the frostiest April in 60 years, it's mid-teen degrees but feels warmer on this windless lunchtime. I stand with my back to Morecambe Bay and look up the arrow-straight canal. It was the conduit for all sorts of industry and raw materials in its heyday. Coal was the chief import to power the businesses, which included shipbuilding, a foundry, sailmakers and a paper mill, amongst others. There is a fascinating 'rolling bridge' that operated from 1881 to 1994. It's now fixed and a public walkway, and also carries an emergency water supply to the adjacent Glaxo (SmithKline) works (although the plant is due to close in 2025). I take some photographs with a bit of difficulty. From whichever angle I try there seems to be a stomach in the way; not mine on this occasion, but a fellow sightseer. He keeps apologising and I keep deleting, till he mooches off to his large camper van. Damn tourists! At the precise moment he leaves, the sun goes in. I retire to the car for lunch - tinned mackerel and peanuts. The view over Morecambe Bay is more satisfying than my protein-fest.

The vista is a wonderful backdrop as I tumble into a post-lunch snooze. To my right the Irish Sea, to the left the viaduct rail crossing over the River Leven Estuary, and straight across is Silverdale and Wharton Sands. Behind me is a pub that's closed for lockdown. But around a table in the dining room, close to the large window overlooking the bay, I can see three large teddy bears and Tigger having a teddy bear's picnic. It brings a smile to the frustrated faces of potential customers who can only gaze in through the window.

The canal is one mile and two furlongs in length - a peculiar measurement until you realize the pub is called The Bay Horse. Travellers would 'rest' here before making the hazardous crossing of the bay by foot, horse or coach. The Romans crossed in AD79, and George Fox, founding father of the Quakers crossed in 1660 on his way to Lancaster prison. JMW Turner crossed on his way back from the Lake District having done sketches for some of his famous paintings - Lancaster Sands and The Old Man of Coniston, for example. In addition, tall ships would call at the pier outside The Bay Horse to collect merchandise on their way to Liverpool, bound for Africa and the slave trade. Dark times these, but overall it's a fascinating, historic spot.

A man arrives in a well-used pickup truck. He rescues a small 'A' frame sign that's blown over and sets it at the side of the road. It says, 'Shrimps' with an arrow pointing along a rough track following the edge of the bay. He lives in a terrific location right by the shore. At least, it's terrific on a beautiful day like today.

I walk to the end of the concrete pier and watch the tide rushing out. It makes an eerie sound as it gurgles and sloshes around the pier-end before heading out to sea. There's a lot of energy going to waste as the River Leven passes by to be dissolved in the Irish Sea. The whole bay is shallow, so that will accentuate the appearance of the rushing water. Quite spooky, really. I make sure the dog is safely on his lead; if he falls in here there would be trouble.

Canal Foot is a jewel.

33

Lost Ladder

I had a preconceived idea that Barrow-in-Furness is a wreck; reasoning based on spurious evidence – namely, because the only person I knew who lived there was himself a wreck. That's slightly unfair. But he was the kind of person who dragged his difficulties around with him. He had a mournful disposition and acted like his horse had died and he was pulling his plough through a claggy field. We first encountered him about ten years ago in Burgundy. His boat was sitting on supports on the quayside. It had been cleaned, surveyed and was awaiting a purchaser. The guy was on board for a couple of days, checking things out.

I was cycling past one morning and heard a shout of anguish, a desperate cry. I feared for someone's safety. Turns out the chap was stuck. Somebody had pinched his ladder, so he was marooned fifteen feet up in the air. I found a spare ladder, rescued him and he sprinted off to the toilet block.

'Bloody Gordon Brown!' he muttered on his return.

I was confused.

'He's knackered the economy, hasn't he?' he grumbled, looking at me with manic eyes. 'Means my boat is worthless. Can't sell the bugger and I can't afford a house even if I do sell it. Bloody politicians.'

His home town was Barrow (maybe still is) and I wanted to see the root of the guy's psychological disarray. On a quick drive through there's lots of prosperous-looking new business. I know historically it's been supremely successful at shipbuilding, not least submarines, which I find fascinating. I remember watching nuclear subs creep out of Holy Lock (near Dunoon on the Clyde) in the early morning mist, each vessel capable of levelling a country. The whole concept gave me the creeps.

I am very impressed with what I can see of Barrow's regeneration; not what I expected at all really. I decide not to look up my old friend. This is only a flying visit and I'd rather leave on a positive note. It's unfortunate that places such as Barrow end up labelled negatively. The fact is that in times past they were thriving, proud communities where the industry was powered by skilled, hard-working people. A person, or a town, shouldn't be looked down on for something that is quite plainly not their fault. Factories, industries, even countries can be manipulated for political or economic reasons. People's lives and livelihoods become the playthings of those holding the aces of power. Folk can be cast down in an instant, but they are no lesser people as a result of their misfortune.

It should be no surprise, therefore, that when they have the chance to thrive again they come back strong. Driving through I can see the metaphorical rubble of the past in the 'weathered' housing and empty, demolished lots where factories and mills once stood, but around the fringes the regeneration is evident and there's new life. That's my impression - I hope I'm right.

* * *

On our way back up north, we find the road we missed earlier and head to Ulverston town centre. Stan Laurel is here in bronze with his old mate and partner. And a dog! I didn't notice the hound during our actual visit, but I spotted it later while reviewing my photos. The poor animal was saddled with the name Laughing Gravy, which is a slang name for booze! Laurel and Hardy played a big part in my childhood. In fact, the further I get from my childhood the more I like them. They remind me of an age of innocence. For me personally it was a time when things were fun and simple and for the world in general when things were less fraught - most importantly, when people had respect for one other. Seeing this wonderful statue brought a smile to my face and a lump to my throat – which distorted my features worse than normal!

What they are is a constant. Whatever the state of play in the world or in our minds, they keep smiling, reminding us that it will all be OK. Their back-catalogue of films sits in our past ready and willing to help us up should we stumble. In a leaflet called *'Stan's Ulverston Town Trail,'* I read that he used to linger while shopping with his Grandma. She'd notice him missing and have to backtrack to rescue her grandson. She'd find him making faces in a shop window. Just add a scratch to the top of the head and you have the basis of a comedic legend. *Whooip di do, whooip di do, di di di do, di di di do.*

Bearing in mind that we're keeping one eye out for a place to live, I asked a friendly lady running her bookstall on the indoor market what the town was like. 'Well, I like it,' she smiled. 'Good job - I've been here sixty years.'

In a nutshell, three reasons there to like a place: indoor market, bookshop and a smiling face. The book I bought was *'British Birds.'* Unfortunately, I'd picked it up from a rack belonging to the stall next door. The lady explained that they looked after each other's stall when one was absent. I felt bad because I'd patronised somebody else when she had been so friendly, so I bought a book from her as well. I'm not made of money, but am a soft-hearted soul. I'll just have to have a little less tripe for supper.

We wandered around the town; it's rather larger than first impressions and we got lost. Couldn't find our way back to the car park. 'Well,' said Jan, 'that's another fine mess ...' Like other places, Ulverston is just awakening from a viral hibernation, so it's rather sparse and difficult to properly appraise. But overall, a welcoming and interesting place, and we'll come back. In fact, so confident are they in Ulverston's enduring popularity that the main photograph on the showcase *Visit Cumbria* website shows the cobbled market square and it's pissing down with rain! Surely they could have picked a better photo, or at least taken one on a day when the sun was shining? Perhaps it never stops raining and they're depicting Ulverston with brutal honesty such that the photo accurately reflects the dire Cumbrian weather. In which case you have to admire their candour – another reason to trust the place and return.

As far as cycling goes around Ulverston, I like the publicity bumf which includes two *'Saunter'* routes. Those sound right up my street ('Right up my disused railway line' doesn't have quite the same ring to it, does it?). Saunters 1 and 2 are both around fourteen miles, which sounds ideal for me and my battery. By contrast there's a route called *'Ladies of the Lakes – The Long One.'* Fifty plus miles, meaning my bike (and me) would run out of juice somewhere around Coniston. I have a tale about Coniston that involves a bicycle and I'm having a shiver at the thought of it. I lost my car keys in the lake …

I went for a swim on one of those rare, roasting hot, early Lake District evenings, not realizing I had the car keys in my shorts pocket. I only discovered my error when we came to leave our little picnic to go and find some accommodation. Car all locked up, my wife and I dressed in shorts and t-shirts. In the days before mobile phones, we asked a passing cyclist to kindly phone the AA on our behalf. It would mean him finding a telephone box (remember them?). We watched him ride off, our fate in his hands, wondering if we might be sleeping in the open air.

The cyclist came good and the AA man duly arrived and pulled our car onto his truck. 'You can get dropped off where you're staying or I can take you home,' he said.

We hadn't got anywhere to stay and we definitely weren't going home, so I asked him to think of another alternative. After a fair degree of huffing and tutting …

'My friend has a garage. I can drop your car there.'

So, he did. On the way he commented that I'd made a bit of a mess of things. I found it hard to argue, but in an attempt at a light-hearted mood-shifter I told him my car keys were at the bottom of Lake Coniston, along with Donald Campbell. There followed a stony silence. Jan and I (she dressed in the AA Man's spare jumper, me in shorts), felt rather conspicuous and grimaced at each other.

'Good friend of mine was Donald Campbell,' said the man quietly.

Oh, Lord! I apologised. Turns out our driver used to work as a mechanic on Bluebird during Sir Donald's water speed record attempts.

We found a room in a B & B. Ironically, it overlooked the pound where our car had been dumped, and I called my brother who would bring up the spare keys the following morning. Lunch on me, I said. Coniston - delightful lake, mixed memories.

We both like Ulverston. We'd only had a couple of hours there but I later find it has two twins. The official one is the French town of Albert in the heart of the site of the Somme battlefields. That is only about ten kilometers from where my wife's uncle is buried, having been killed on the first day of the battle of the Somme in July 1916. I think we'll be taking time to visit Albert when circumstances allow. The second twinning is in friendship with Harlem, Georgia, the birthplace of Oliver Hardy. This was only arranged recently, in 2016, when it was voted for overwhelmingly by the councillors of Ulverston. To me it just seems an appropriate way to celebrate the lives of two men who came together by chance and gave the world so much joy. Diamonds from a golden age.

34

I'll come back another time

I am aware that some people in this neck of the Cumbrian woods have dual careers / incomes. For example, I came across a garden maintenance man who also delivered livestock. On weekends in June, when I met him, he delivered young pheasants, thousands of them, to shooting estates as far away as mid-Scotland. Hill farming is a tough way to make a living. It's not easy to cajole a decent livelihood from the land, and it can be a precarious business having to rely on weather and market fluctuations, so people supplement their income however they can.

Another double-income person appears to be the cycle shop proprietor whose shop only opens between 3.00 PM to 7.00 PM, Monday to Saturday. Except Wednesdays, when it doesn't open at all. I'm making a presumption here that they do have another business that delays the shop opening, as opposed to just being late sleepers.

I made two visits. First, on Tuesday morning to find it didn't open till the afternoon. Second, on Friday afternoon when I was sure it would be open. I was tingling with anticipation at the prospect of buying some oil for my bicycle chain. However, I was met with a supplementary sign, pinned on top of the regular sign that advised us of the limited opening hours. This second sign told me that the shop was completely closed for a week.

I do find this peculiar because the town is awash with bikes. Surely there is good business to be had. Not only is Kirkby Stephen on the official 'Coast to Coast' route (between St. Bees on the west coast to Robin Hood's Bay in the east), there are also many other lovely rides in the area. I'm probably just a bit ratty because I couldn't get any oil. I even enquired in the town's main supermarket, the Co-op. A helpful lady didn't think they did chain oil but told me all the oils they stocked were down aisle 3. Needless to say, neither sunflower nor olive were really what I was after.

Despite the lack of oil, I've been out on the bike a lot. Incidentally, you can improvise if you're without oil. I recall a friend who lost all the oil out of his gearbox on his boat. Having no spare oil he shoved two bananas in the gearbox, which gave them enough lubrication to reach the next port. I kid you not.

Anyhow, the sun is shining and I've swapped my nasty, glo-green cycling top for a bright yellow gilet, the type road-menders wear with reflective strips. In fact, it is a road-mender's waistcoat! Gone, too, are the long pants. Instead, I wear a pair of mountain-biker shorts - the type of thing footballers wore in the 1920s; masses of material and voluminous, but with pockets. In fact, I look rather like Don Estelle (Lofty) from '*It Ain't Half Hot Mum.*'

My legs are like seasoned teak and my toned buttocks rock solid, like two halves of an underripe peach. I should really be the envy of all those I encounter. Not that they really give a damn; most of them just go on eating grass and baaing. However, legs and bum is where the good bits end. Above there is a stomach like semi-set jelly in a bin bag and, higher still, a couple of chins resembling an ill-fitting roll-neck sweater. These flobbery accessories have developed despite a pretty reasonable diet. It's the peripherals that are doing the damage, like red wine and peanuts.

I refer to the wine because I recently rode past an 'establishment of temperance' in Kirby Stephen. Being somebody that enjoys a glass or two of the red stuff, anything with the word temperance in it gives me withdrawal symptoms. The Temperance Hall was built in 1856 to service the needs of those who had 'taken the pledge'; this at a time when there were supposedly 17 pubs and inns in the town – and it's not that big a place. But the temperance movement was determined and it did make a difference - alcohol did play a big part in domestic and social unrest.

There is no unrest in our house, thank goodness, but I felt peculiar gazing upon the temperance hall - light-headed, heart thumping. It was a similar feeling to the one I recall on one occasion in the heart of France. We'd moored the barge in a lovely spot in the shade of some plane trees on a riverbank. A wonderful photo opportunity had presented itself. Overlooking the scene was a substantial hill topped by a church; a position from where I would be able to get a panoramic photo of our boat in an idyllic setting. So, I cycled all the way up the hill. Even in my lowest gear it took quite a while, and it proved much further than I thought.

When I finally got there, I was not only totally knackered, I also couldn't see the boat because it was hidden behind a stand of trees part way down the hill. It was a very warm day and I was feeling a bit light-headed, so I went to sit in the shade of the church doorway to cool off.

'Ca va?' asked a kindly official wearing ecclesiastical robes. 'Are you OK?'

I was ashen-faced and my heart was thudding. He looked alarmed when I gently thumped my chest and asked if they were open for funerals. He smiled and walked off, probably thinking, 'Bloody foreigners.'

This day I was showing signs of wear. Looking back, it was another sign of my gradual deterioration but at the time not drastic enough to realize there was something amiss. I never used to worry about hills and I'm sure I used to recover quicker. In fact, I'd count 'recovery time' in minutes rather than weeks.

I remember cycling with my mate from Church Stretton to Shrewsbury on the A49 trunk road. It was back in the mid-1970s when we were in our teens and we'd have been as fit as we ever would be. But even so, this day was a test. There was a howling wind straight into us and it was lashing down. Fourteen miles into the teeth of a gale would test anyone. This was in the days when that particular road was safe to cycle, when there were many fewer cars and lorries. Today, there's no way I would tackle it. It was a frightening enough experience in a car last time I was down there, never mind on a bike.

Anyway, me and my mate were having a real battle. We were on the way to his parents' house on the outskirts of Shrewsbury, where we'd find food and shelter. We'd take turns leading. Each time we passed one another we'd whisper, in time with our pedaling, 'cup of tea and a piece of cake, cup of tea and a piece of cake.' Although the promise of a restorative induced us to greater endeavours, we did have to stop a couple of times because we were laughing so much.

35

Up The Dales

We leave Cumbria and enter Richmondshire. I didn't even know there WAS a Richmondshire. Nevertheless, I'm delighted to be here. The name has an old-world feel. Perhaps even an other-world feel, maybe somewhere you'd come across in Hobbit-land. Though it sounds like it, it's not actually a county - it's an administrative centre covering a large area of North Yorkshire. One place it administers is Hawes, the town we're aiming for (specifically, the Wensleydale cheese factory and, more importantly, the shop).

We have the dog with us. He's learned a couple of new tricks during our northern stay. Firstly, to avoid sheep, which is marvellous. Secondly, to vomit in the car, which is less marvellous. So, tingling with anticipation at the prospect of perusing a regal assortment of cheese, we discover he's ralphed in the back of the car. An enthusiasm-dampening happening, if ever there is one. We can't blame him. Jan certainly doesn't; she blames me for driving on twisty roads. I don't think that's very fair; I had little option. If I'd driven in a straight line I'd have been through fields and rivers. She nobly offers to have a tidy-up while I go shopping. As unfortunate incidents go, it's not too bad, really - just a few biscuits.

I banter with the cheesemonger. He's dressed in a very smart, all-white cheesemongery outfit, including hat. We're from rival counties and the Lancashire / Yorkshire war is still being fought in isolated but intense pockets.

I am able to be rather more forthright than he. He has to be careful because he's at the very forefront of the Wensleydale Cheese operation. As such he can't say anything unseemly for fear of damaging their reputation – which is very, very good internationally, as well as here at home.

When he'd soaked up my witty, verbal punches, uppercuts and jabs that would have felled a lesser mortal, he was very helpful and knowledgeable. I end up with a shopping bag full of goodies, including four different cheeses. Among others, I've chosen a 'Gold' one and another run through with cranberries. My mouth waters as I record these words and I'm tempted to go and open a bottle of port and have myself a major treat. But, best not - I'll wait till I've had breakfast.

I've spent a goodly sum and Jan has a look in my bag when I return to the car. She looks to make sure she doesn't double up when she goes in for her dose of retail therapy. Actually, she buys some delicious herby biscuits and some more cheese - then reveals they are to give away to friends! Sacrilege.

We've parked on a car park about two hundred yards down a steep hill. One hour. But now we decide to take advantage of the open air café and have brunch. It's a pristine landscape with a backdrop of the fells beyond the River Ure. There's still nearly half an hour left on the parking ticket. We wait ten minutes (which is quite a long time when absolutely nothing is happening) and finally a lady arrives with the menus.

'We'd like two coffees and I'll have a cheese toastie, please,' says Jan. 'Made with Wensleydale cheese,' she added with a big smile - her attempt at a cross-border ice-breaker.

'I'll send Julie over to take your order.'

It sounded like coping with our order was above the waitress's pay grade. Perhaps she wasn't an official waitress; instead, maybe she was specifically employed as a menu-deliverer. She was a mature, well-spoken lady and appeared perfectly capable of writing down our simple order (or even just remembering it) and conveying our modest requests to the kitchen, so it was all a little surprising.

A further ten minutes later Julie hadn't appeared so I decided to go and extend the parking ticket. I just had the feeling that we'd get nabbed by the

Hawes Traffic Patrolman. I forgot to take the car key with me so had to tuck the supplementary ticket externally, in the window rubber. I was reticent about leaving it vulnerable to an opportunist ticket-thief, this being the land of sheep rustlers and carpetbagging Tykes. The situation was ripe for my ticket being pinched and us being fined for overtime.

I got back to the café and Julie (fully-trained waitress) had been. Jan had lost her appetite so she'd just ordered two coffees. They had obviously arrived just as I'd left because mine was now stone-cold. I could tell it had probably, at one time, been quite an appealing brew because the creamy froth looked delicious; the sort of thing you could have photographed and put in a magazine such as *Yorkshire Life*. Unfortunately, it had set into a sort of milky glue and I had a bit of a job getting to the liquid part underneath - much to the amusement of the man sitting at the next table, who looked down and pretended to read a map when he realized I'd spotted him.

I frowned a mock frown at him, a frown with minimal impact because I was covered in gooey froth. That made Jan smile, too. I told the man, mock-pointedly, that it was nice to encounter someone with a sense of humour, even if he was taking advantage of someone else's misfortune. I'd seen him arrive in a sports car, so we talked about his old MG. He was trundling around Yorkshire with his wife. It was a grand old thing (the car, not the wife), an MGB I think, with the roof down. The problem is with these old things is that by the time you can afford one you're too inflexible to get in and out of the damn thing. He told me they had toured Belgium in it before the virus hit. I told him we had lived there for a while and I was always moved and in awe of the memorial reminders of the World Wars. His wife piped up for the first time at this point, telling us that she couldn't stand Flanders - uninteresting, boring place. Time to go before I said something I'd regret.

We had a mooch round Hawes town because we had time left on the parking ticket. It was busy with people doing the same as us – mooching. Some had bemused expressions, like us, wondering what sort of creative thinking had arrived at the prices in the succession of antique shops. There were also clothing shops selling some very nice country gear. I spotted an enormous pair of thick knee-length socks, just the things to cope with my diabetic feet in winter. I would have bought them, but the shop was shut. Darn it (oh dear!).

The Dales are a rather different prospect to where we're staying in the Howgills. It's more reflective of the real world somehow, in that it's noticeably busier and more 'commercial.' I get the feeling that people want to squeeze you a bit, get out of you what they can. I can understand this entirely; folk have to make a living, particularly after the difficult times we've lived through recently. I can accept the premium prices because it's all set in stunning countryside and lovely looking towns and villages. It's a peculiar paradox that we're drawn to the most wonderful place to be somewhat exploited.

* * *

We're travelling roughly southwest, heading for Ingleton, another famous Dales town. We're just coming out of another lockdown, so people are desperate for a bit of freedom and it appears that half the population has arrived at Ribblehead Viaduct. It really is an iconic sight in the sunshine. It brings to life the world-famous images of steam trains on the Settle / Carlisle run passing over Batty Moss in the Ribble Valley.

As we approach there are conservatively a hundred cars and vans parked up near the viaduct. Off to the right we can see distant hang-gliders sky-sailing over Whernside mountain, the highest of Yorkshire's 'three peaks.' Beyond that, Cumbria. I have a job taking a photo of the viaduct without the real world interfering - cars, vans, etc. There are hundreds of folks enjoying the wonderful scenery hereabout; walking, hand-gliding, photographing or just out enjoying the sunshine. It's wonderful to see people free of the virus' shackles. Although the moors are enormous and there is plenty of space, I can see people on the distant hills like tiny ants on their hill. The busyness is a change for me because where I've been walking and cycling recently I'm hard pushed to see five people a day.

One thing I notice are the incredible dry stone walls that quarter the landscape. They start on the valley floor and run right to the top of the Whernside Ridge, about three kilometers from the viaduct. Many are arrow-straight and building them would have taken endless hours of back-bent graft. The hills here are rolling and gentle. The Howgills next door are slightly 'lumpier,' described by the wonderful Mr Wainwright in his guide as like a herd of sleeping elephants. Further west is the Lake District proper where the hills are far more severe and dramatic. It's all beautiful in its own way; we're lucky to have it.

Ingleton deserves more time than we can spare today, so we avail ourselves of the lavatorial facilities in the Tourist Information Centre (it's rare to find one open at the moment) and head toward iconic Kirkby Lonsdale. But not before we've seen Ingleton Viaduct. Sadly, it's fenced off and doesn't carry trains, or bikes or even walkers. What the viaduct does carry is a high speed … wait for it … fibre-optic cable, installed by local volunteers to enable the village to have a decent broadband connection; a means of communication through which they can promote their viaduct that nobody can walk on.

As viaducts go it's, well, like any other to be frank, and somehow it seems rather a waste of an historic memorial to a bygone railway. To be fair, we have been spoilt because we've travelled the Pontcysyllte Aqueduct on the Llangollen Canal, which is longer, higher, older and still in regular use. We've also just come past Ribblehead Viaduct, which is as impressive as viaducts get.

As we're walking back to the car, there's a sign off to the left: 'No Caravans.' The sign points down a steep hill and at the bottom is a field, stuffed full of caravans. We leave with a feeling that Ingleton probably has more to offer than our brief skirmish.

Kirkby Lonsdale is one of those 'honey pot' towns - an icon and flagship of Yorkshire Dales tourism. And it's busy. For me this is a place to visit at 5.30 AM on my bike while everyone else is asleep. Now, mid-afternoon on a weekday, it's heaving. It's a working town, a tourism hotspot and filled to overflowing because school is just coming out.

There's a 'craft' market where there's a chap selling gin, presumably locally made. I hear him say, in a particularly non-Yorkshire accent, 'I'm only here for a bit of brand-awareness.' He was trying to impress a lady with a red setter. Not very Yorkshire market stall speak either, if you ask me. It sounded like he hadn't sold much, probably because his product was pricey and aimed at the

Range Rover brigade, not the likes of me and most of the other day-trippers who'd had a job finding somewhere to park in addition to having a limited budget.

Apart from gin man, there were other stalls with some lovely stuff for sale, including woodwork, artwork and clothes - none of which we needed. But the afternoon was rescued beautifully because I found a stall selling hog-roast pork. I have a very sensitive hooter and was drawn in from some distance. The pork is the produce of a local farmer, and boy did his little corner of Kirkby Lonsdale smell good. I don't eat bread, so I asked for a tray of succulent pork with a big lump of crackling. I sat on a bench outside a pub and watched the beautiful people glide by. They glance over (some with envy, some with alarm) as I chomp my pork and crunch my crackling. Proper grub!

Designer dogs share the space with lugubrious, chunky Labradors - the difference between status and class right there. Now, at school's out time, the high street is gridlocked with expensive cars, many of them 4 x 4s. Despite the pork, this place is not for me. It's a lovely old town but it's coated in a blingy, expensive veneer, quite out of keeping with the natural, rolling landscape that is the wonderful Yorkshire Dales. You can tell I'm an outdoor chap, can't you?

36

Elfstadentocht

Friesland, a province in northwest Netherlands, is host to a race called the *Elfstedentocht*. Literal translation: Eleven Cities Tour. It is a race of almost 200 kilometers, where speed skaters travel the frozen canals passing through eleven towns and 'cities,' starting and finishing in Leeuwarden. Competitors have a card stamped in each town as proof that they visited. The race can only be held when there is a sufficient depth of ice, around 15 cm, so it has not been run for a number of years. Climate change is getting in the way of the creation of new heroes.

Thin ice means no skating, but there are other ways to do the tour, including cycling. The route is a bit longer, at 235 km, and the 'official' tour is limited to 15,000 cyclists (only!). I mistakenly got wrapped up in it. We'd moored our boat just outside a little town called Sloten and I cycled in to investigate why the lift bridge was out of commission. Me and my second-hand (at least) machine got tangled up with a flood of riders who were passing through, queuing to have their cards stamped. The Elfstedentocht (cycling version) was in town. It's actually an incredible sight - multi-thousands of people of all shape and size on a staggering array of different machinery.

Some were obviously very serious riders with expensive-looking accessories, sleek bikes and exposed bits glistening with a healthy sheen. Others obviously had a more relaxed approach - not that you can get too relaxed when completing a ride of this length. I came across one chap slumped against a tree trying to get his body going again. 'Just 60 kilometers to go,' he gasped. I looked around for an ambulance, just in case.

I'd ridden about 300 metres from the boat on my 40-Euro equipment (that had developed a worrying rattle and squeak within the last couple of days). I stood out like a sore thumb, which wasn't helped by the fact that I was going against the flow. I was making my way in search of lunch, specifically the mobile fish and chip shop doing good business in a car park. I was 'competitor' number 15,001 and the only cyclist not wearing a helmet and the only one going backwards. Among the low-level chatter of people swapping tales of derring-do, a porky entity attached to a nagging squeak eased by, not entirely unnoticed, on the periphery. Would they know I was an outsider just by looking? Or worse, English? Damn right they would. Such is the prestige in which cycling is held here, I was like the streaker at an international rugby match - without certain compensating attributes.

By midday, the cycles had all passed through and I'd had my lunch, so we anticipated making some progress before the day was out. But then the peace was shattered. It was the turn of the motorcycles. The bridge operator had taken lunch and returned to his control booth. There was a revving, clattering roar as the barrier was raised and a mixture of modern and classic bikes made a terrific racket as they powered over the bridge. To be honest, it was fascinating and I saw some very impressive machinery. I was told there were only around a thousand motorbikes. Only.

* * *

Though some rides are quite short, they can be important. One tiddler I undertook allowed me to tick off Germany as another country visited on my lifetime list. To be honest, it was a semi-accident. I didn't realize I'd left the Netherlands till I saw a sign saying '*Achtung*' (Danger) warning me of a mucky ditch. I checked my map and, sure enough, here I was, creeping along the outskirts of Europe's powerhouse. I bought a chocolate bar in a petrol station as proof of my visit. I spotted later, printed on the back, 'Made in the UK.'

Another quickie was to Amsterdam. 'Quickie' is perhaps not the best way to describe a visit to the self-styled 'sex capital of the world.' I was swept into town on a tsunami of bikes, workers surfing into the city at the start of the day. To be honest it was rather disconcerting traveling at 15 kph being part of something fluid and alive. I was riding the rapids and didn't really feel in full control as we traversed roundabouts and swooped through an underpass. As we reached what I presumed was the center, or business district perhaps, people just peeled off and in no time I was on a bridge over a small, tree-lined canal with just a few locals for company; perhaps the odd tourist too, maybe even the occasional person looking to pay for a good time, despite the early hour.

It's a leafy, cobbled world built around canals. The muted colours are reminiscent of a painting by an old Dutch Master. Even the shops look somehow rustic, their autumn colours blending in with the streets and waterways. I see my bike leaning on a bridge as I back off to take a photo, and to be honest it looks like a bit of a sad relic. It could easily be the property of a sad old git who's gone to avail himself of the 'local services.'

The Netherlands really is a mixture of then and now. They are ultra-high-tech and innovative with their national flood defenses; a quarter of the country is below sea-level, after all. Some of their engineering is stunning and fearless. Then they are also wonderful at maintaining their traditional culture, particularly through festivals. We visited one celebrating historic ships, for example. It was a magnificent spectacle. The pride that both boat-owners and visitors showed for these stunning vessels was plain to see.

On one occasion, while cruising our knackered old barge, we had to merge onto the mighty River Waal for a few kilometers. It's one of three big rivers we had to traverse in order to get from The Netherlands to France. And this one is big. We'd moored a few kilometers short of the river in a quiet bird-tweeting nature reserve, so I went to investigate on my bike. I was glad I was disguised (helmet, sunglasses) because when I saw this mighty river for the first time my heart thudded into my boots. I must have gone white as a sheet. It was enormous - a light-brown muddy serpent flowing left to right at about four kilometers an hour. I stood there astride my bike wondering what the hell we were letting ourselves in for. Huge, multi-thousand-tonne ships thundered by. The following day we would be among them. It was either that or turn round and go back north. If I thought cycling into Amsterdam was worrying, this was in a whole other league. Ultimately, I don't like going back.

I rode back to the boat almost in a state of shock. I don't know if Gorinchem is a nice place because I cycled through it in a blur. I had to decide how much to tell Jan. How honest should I be? Ultimately, I was economical. Had I told her my true feelings our adventure would have ended right there. Doing something for the first time is invariably the best. That boat experience on the Waal was very nerve-wracking. Our boat was a shrimp compared to the commercial monsters servicing the needs of Western European commerce. Most boating is a real pleasure and we are usually able to avoid big out-of-our-depth waterways. Imaging cycling on a concrete-walled motorway among cars and trucks - that's what our Waal experience felt like. Of course, on a bike we can avoid motorways (indeed are obligated to) because there is always an alternative.

* * *

I don't cycle as fast as some, nor go as far, but that doesn't stop me getting a buzz out of it. As I've said before, if you get nervous (or outright frightened) about something, you know you're alive. There's a real buzz getting through something you're anxious about. Generally, riding a bike over an unknown route can be wonderful. I love to go on mystery tours. In my youth it was full throttle, highest, steepest. Nowadays I go at a pace where I miss less, certainly the first time I tackle a route. I'm so glad I was able to hear and see a curlew for the first time; I was quiet so it was close. I've paused, still and silent for a moment, to look a roe deer in the eye.

Jan had a 'moment' in Belgium, Diksmuide to be precise, where we were living temporarily. It's a god-fearing, wealthy town. Clean, prosperous and 'reassuringly expensive' as the advert goes. The price of a pack of underwear here would buy me a pretty reasonable sports jacket back home. Mind, I never was the most sartorially gifted. On this occasion, coming up to Christmas, there was an evening sales special on where many shops opened late and had rails of clothes out on the pavements. It's something they do from time to time and a good idea - like a Belgian Black Friday. It's also a convivial time where people meet and chat (more than usual) on the cobbled streets and the large central square.

Jan was on her trusty (slightly rusty) donated bicycle 'of a certain age.' She was perusing a rail of clothes while still sitting on her bike, passing the time of day and muttering appreciatively with a couple of local ladies on the opposite side of the rail. Nothing took Jan's fancy, despite the big price drops, so she moved away. Unfortunately, one item of clothing had got trapped in the bike so as she moved off, the whole rail went with her – much to the surprise of the two lady shoppers who were rooting for a bargain on the other side.

37

Gone West

I set off for another little tour, a house-hunting scouting venture. It's really just to confirm we can't afford to live anywhere I've actually heard of. It's a clear day, crisp and clean; in fact, the air is so pure that the clouds look like representations of what I imagine they should look like. They are so clearly defined against the blue sky they look like artist's impressions.

Then, out of the blue, a double decker bus. I've been hereabouts for the best part of a month (spread over a number of visits) and have never seen any sort of bus, never mind a vintage double decker. It's one of the Cumbria Classic Coaches fleet and the board on the front says it's on its way from Barnard Castle via Kirkby Stephen, but it's empty. Then it turns off into a farmyard that looks like a vehicle graveyard and the romance goes out of the moment. Besides, had it carried on along this road there's a low bridge not far ahead. Had the bus hit that at any speed it would have taken out the Settle Carlisle railway line. Like our boating days, expect the unexpected.

I'm heading for rugby league territory. I know both Whitehaven and Workington have great rugby credentials but know little else about the towns, other than they are on the Cumbrian west coast so have probably been visited by a long-haired Scottish TV presenter on his way round the British coastline. Whitehaven is not far north of Barrow, the extent of my last scouting expedition.

I travel straight through the Lake District via Keswick, scene of one of my indiscretions in about 1980. I got sacked by the hotel where I was working as a barman for 'fraternising with the guests.' What do you visualize seeing that phrase? Well, you're wrong! What happened was an Indian man and wife came to stay and they were racially abused by our head waitress. She was a feisty old trout at the best of times but on this occasion, as far as I was concerned, she'd gone way too far. I felt really sorry for the Indian couple who were lovely, gentle people. I could see they were upset when they came back to the bar after dinner and explained what had happened. So, I bought them a drink, then they bought me one back and ...

At closing time, I bought a bottle of malt out of stock and we took it back to my room. This is bad form apparently, probably because the staff accommodation was four star and the hotel rooms only two! Anyhow, the hotel owner came charging in to investigate the noise and he and I had a 'heated' discussion which resulted in me seeking alternative employment. Shortly after I left, the hotel closed; it simply didn't have the same class after I'd gone. It is now a nursing home.

I bypass Keswick, just in case the 'wanted' posters are still out, and arrive in Whitehaven. And what a pleasant surprise it is. I am really, really impressed by the harbour area and, being a naturally boat-loving person, spend a fabulous hour wandering around. The inner port area is divided up by substantial, original harbour walls, and now plays host to Whitehaven Marina. It is a real gem.

There's an elderly guy sitting on a bench overlooking the harbour. He looks at peace and relaxed in the bright sun so I decide to go and wreck his morning. We agree that it's a nice day and the port looks lovely; I ask him if he lives here and, if so, what the town is like. Turns out he retired here a few years ago and lives 'up yonder,' pointing to a bank of white-rendered houses up the hillside to the north. He tells me he comes down to the port every morning and enjoys watching the world go by for an hour. If this guy were an advert for Whitehaven the place would be thriving; his enthusiasm is infectious and he obviously loves the place.

I wander round the port and look at the pincers that comprise the outer harbour walls. There's a lock between the outer and inner port areas. Today is beautiful, but I can imagine winter storms lashing this west-facing coast when sea-farers would need all the protection going. There are many boats in the harbour from pleasure yachts to cruisers and fishing boats. Not many fishing boats.

West Cumbria and coal mining were synonymous and here in Whitehaven there's a wonderful memorial to the men and women who worked in the mining industry, a trade that played a huge part in the history of the town. Whitehaven's last mine, Haig Pit, closed in 1986 although they are currently trying to open a new undersea pit to mine coke. The memorial, incorporating four people round a large block of coal, depicts a miner, a deputy, a brigadesman (mine rescue specialist) and a screen lass. Screen lasses were women who worked at sorting and breaking the coal. Back-breaking graft, prompting one person who witnessed them to say, 'They don't want lasses working there, they want horses.' It's an amazing sculpture, unveiled in 2005 by a former screen lass. Part of the engraving on the plaque says, *'In celebration of the past, to inform the present and encourage the future.'* This is not the first town in West Cumbria where I've felt the pride the residents have in their heritage.

Just down the coast is St. Bees. Not sure I didn't play school sport against them at one point, but the memory's a bit misty. But St. Bees marks the start of a 'coast to coast' walk. My (nearly) son-in-law recently led a walk which ends in Robin Hood's Bay, near Whitby. This was his first 'crossing' as a Mountain Leader, guiding six guests the 190 miles over two weeks. Judging by the progress reports that reached base camp, it went really well.

I sense more history as I look out at the watchtower (erected around 1730 on the outer harbour wall) and the old pier. I hesitate to go into the town proper because I don't want to spoil the feel-good factor of the harbour, but I vow to come back.

By comparison, Workington a little further north looks tired. Despite there being some new development, it looks like what its name used to suggest - a working town, but on the verge of retirement. Numerous, white-rendered council houses in blocks of twos and fours looked down on a harbour that hints at better days. But wait a minute. It's totally unfair to label a place on a drive-through. It's trying to regenerate after a hugely successful past. For example, if you travel by train in the UK, there's a good chance the track you're on was made in Workington. They had a massive steel and smelting industry. Let's hope it thrives again. I leave on a high after a very pleasant young lass working the harbourside shop sold me some peanuts for my lunch.

* * *

Maryport today is a new town built on the rubble of Roman occupation. Previously called Ellenfoot, it was redeveloped by local landowner Humphrey Senhouse who named his new town and harbour after his wife, Port – joking! Mary, of course. It was a wealthy place built on shipbuilding and coal. Fletcher Christian of Bounty fame lived nearby, and the harbour and lighthouse featured in L.S. Lowry's paintings. Much of the town's history is depicted on a wonderful feature called the Alauna (the Roman name for the town) Aura.

I'm just scratching the surface of this coastline but I like it. North of Maryport, heading up towards Silloth, the coastline changes dramatically. It's far less hilly and for much of the route the road is separated from the Solway Firth by sand dunes. Almost all available space is full of camper vans and cars. It's all very open, looking like a retirement haven to be honest, with lovely views over the estuary. There's also plenty of flat territory for cycling. My metaphorical ears prick up at cycling potential. I'm heading for Silloth, partly because I played golf there many years ago and want another look, and partly because I'm told it's a nice safe town.

I stop for lunch on the estuary front near Allonby, where I park on a wide grassy common. Before me is a coastal path, then the estuary. I'm looking out towards Mount Criffel (which is more of a hill, to be honest) in Dumfries and Galloway. But it's a fabulous view on a windless, sunny day. The weather has brought people flocking, particularly old people who don't like hills, and also people who've been locked down for what feels like years. I eat my peanuts and live the dream.

I'm parked next to an old Jaguar inhabited by a man and woman. Their windows are open, which is an obvious invitation for me to ruin their lunch.

They are a very well-spoken couple, of some age, and he tells me it is their first time out for months. I tell them I am just doing a bit of touring and tell them where I've been, including seeing Stan and Ollie in Ullswater and having lunch at Canal Foot. He looks at me with interest as if to say, 'Mm, lunch at the Bay Horse, Canal Foot. You're a lucky guy. You must have more cash than you appear to have!' (Admittedly, I was dressed for pleasure, not business). Then I tell him the pub was shut so I had a tin of mackerel and some peanuts in the car, followed by a snooze. They both laugh politely.

With a bit of prompting, he tells me they live close to Lancaster and the M6 motorway near Forton Service Station. He says they have recently opened a Marks and Spencer within the service station. 'Fortunate for us,' he says, 'because having an M&S within walking distance of your home enhances the value, and it's a good selling point.' I find this pretty funny and wonder whether there is actually access to the Services without going down the motorway. But I keep quiet; I don't want to spoil his story. I do ask what would happen should the M&S close down for any reason - would he market the property as *'being within walking distance of Forton Service Station'*? He has to concede that his marketing strategy hangs by a thread. I like this chap and tell him that our house in Littleborough has an inside lavatory, a rarity in our part of the world. That, I tell him, is the main talking point round where we live.

Silloth on Solway is not as I remember it; the golf course entrance is hidden away behind an industrial estate. The town? Well, I don't remember that at all. Maybe I never looked last time. Perhaps I came, fired a few golf balls into the estuary, then left again. I used to be singularly focussed, unaware that there was a world beyond the golf links. But today I'm on a (half-hearted) mission to answer the question, 'Could I live here?'

First, it's packed. School holidays, I think. Lots of kids, cars and camper vans on an estuary-front green. It's a large communal area being well used. The town is spread out; there's more space between houses and wider roads than most places I've been. It feels like Silloth melted after it was built and everything oozed out a bit, taking advantage of its isolation and spreading out.

I've reached a low point in my journey (twenty feet above sea level, according to my telephone's altimeter), so I console myself with a few peanuts. I'm near the start of Hadrian's Wall but it's not working; there's a family of Scots parked next to me. Lockdown has sort of eased but I'm not sure whether they are illegal day-trippers. I don't challenge them because they have a big dog and two fiery children, any of whom could see me off.

It's a wide-street place, with lots of openness and sea air. Somewhere where I can spread my arms and sing gaily. If I tried that back home they'd probably lock me up.

During the return to base camp, I ask myself could I live up on this coast? Tell you what, there's just something about being by the sea.

38

As Graveyards go.....

Another day we look closer to home. Sedbergh is dominated by a public school and a lovely old church. It reinvented itself as England's book-town, following the model of Hay-on-Wye, which hosts its world-famous literary festival. I wondered whether Hay would be discombobulated (good literary word) because Sedbergh has taken the 'England's Book-Town' title. Then, showing literary ignorance, I discover that Hay is actually in Wales - but only by about an inch on my map, so I was close.

Sadly, just about all Sedbergh's shops are closed due to the lockdown, a pity because I enjoy a good peruse of the written word. I like to roam among the tomes and grovel among the novels. Instead, we go and investigate the fabulous old Norman church. We can't get in here either. Seems the good Lord doesn't want to catch anything, so we take a stroll round the graveyard. It seems rather a waste of a parking fee; we could have walked round a graveyard back home - after all, they are all pretty similar. However, this one overlooked the sports field of the famous old school, so at least those at rest do have a wonderful view. I flash up images of boys in uniform being ordered around by their seniors and spanked. I should know; I went to such a school in the 1970s.

Tending a flowerbed in the graveyard is a local chap, a friendly sort who extols the virtues of the town and the famous parents of some of the kids. He is upbeat despite not being able to afford anywhere to live in his own town. He is currently looking for somewhere to rent and I get the feeling that if he's successful it will be because of the benevolence of someone he knows. Market rates here for purchase or rent are high and steepling, as townies realize they would rather come and ruin a rural way of life than live cheek by jowl in an urban scrum while being coughed on.

I look out wistfully over the manicured cricket field and recall my own sporting days. I was lucky enough to be captain of the school cricket team. (I wasn't awfully good, there was just no one else prepared to do it - in one lad's case because he wanted to concentrate on A-Level studies. I thought at the time he'd got his priorities all skewed, which is probably why I sell a few books and he's running a large pharmaceutical concern.) When we won a cricket match we'd have an illicit beer and cigarette in the showers. If we lost we'd get thrashed with a belt! Happy days. Not the same nowadays, of course. It wouldn't be ale and ciggies, it would be Red Bull and designer skunk. And it wouldn't be the belt, it would be counselling.

There's a memorial stone on the main road through the town. Quite an impressive little stone structure, actually. Rather ornate for what it is. It commemorates the fact the road was widened for Queen Victoria's Diamond Jubilee. I have to say I never realized she'd put so much weight on.

* * *

Appleby is another place we want to have a look at. Bear in mind we are still looking for potential places to live, should we decide on a change of direction. Appleby is famous, not least, for its horse fair. This has the reputation of being an occasion when gypsies and travellers ride horses around the town and cavort in the River Eden. There must be more to it than that, so I investigate a little. I discover that the fair is under the governance of ... wait for it: *The Appleby Horse Fair Multi-Agency Strategic Co-ordinating Group.* I suspect the primary requirement for joining the group would be to remember it's complicated name and have the ability to repeat it without referring to notes. Virus-dependent, hopefully this year's fair will go ahead in August (it's currently April).

It's a massive event, billed as the biggest traditional gypsy fair in Europe, known among the traveling communities as akin to a huge family get-together. One tradition is the washing of the horses in the river (not cavorting!) then parading them through the town. Originally this was done through the lanes and streets, but as the fair became more popular and attracted more participants and tourists it became increasingly dangerous, so they created *The Flashing Lane* which is a 'run' through the centre of the fair where things could be better controlled. Horses are paraded both for show and as a marketplace where buyers can get a good look at the animals on offer. Some will be bred for pure speed, others to pull wagons; the latter will need a good temperament, strength and stamina.

Having briefly encountered a few ponies close up in their natural environment on the fells, I have the urge to go and see the Appleby Fair. Despite the fact that horses in general terrify me.

We're seeing all these towns and villages through blinkers, or through a mist. They are not bustling as they would normally be because most of the shops are closed. All we can do is get an idea of what they're about. There are no horses in Appleby but lots of daffodils which seem resistant to Covid. We sit quietly by the River Eden and listen to the ghosts of excited, busier times.

Appleby's main street, which is wide, has been described as one of the most impressive in England. This is one of those claims about which little can be substantiated. Who described it thus? The person who wrote the tourist blurb? The company that resurfaced the road? It is nice, I admit, but we'll have to revisit in a non-viral era to see just how good it really is. Perhaps we'll come during the horse fair when a mountain of horse poop may just add that little extra.

In Appleby, Jan found 'the perfect handbag' in the window of a little shop right next to the river bridge. Sadly for her (but gladly for our bank balance) it was shut, but was 'opening up again whenever possible.' Well, we returned three months later and Jan got her bag. While she shopped I walked along the river. Close by to my left is Appleby Cricket Club; in fact, only a low fence separates the outfield from the river path. I bade good morning to a man gathering rope from round the field's boundary. Those were the last two words I would utter for about fifteen minutes as the chap set off on a stream of consciousness dialogue unleashed from eighteen months of no-contact lockdown.

Actually, he was full of enthusiasm for his beloved club and very interesting. He told me the extent of various floods the club had endured, one of which, in 2015 I believe, left the whole field four feet under River Eden water. They have since had various grants to improve the ground and build a new pavilion (on stilts) but have barely had chance to use their upgraded facilities because of Covid. The day we chat (or he did), the weather is idyllic and we can both imagine the strike of bat on ball and ripples of applause. We are two avid cricket fans imagining an archetypal English scene played out before us.

When I finally get a word in I tell him I have to leave because our car park ticket is due to expire. I explain that we'd been gifted the ticket by a nice lady who was returning home early because her son had been sick on the swings. It would be ironic if we got charged a penalty for a ticket we'd been given. The man smiled but probably thought I was a tight-fisted Lancastrian git come to plunder his town. I pointed out that we had spent cash locally on coffees in a community centre, buoying the economy to the tune of a fiver. I wished him well and told him that I hoped his cricket club would soon thrive again. We parted as friends.

39

Who's the Imposter?

I don't know when I'll be back, so the dog and I take a last walk to our number one favourite spot. We set off at five in the morning just as the sun is making an impression, kissing the fell-tops, turning them the colour of honey. I tell the sleepy-eyed dog that the sooner we leave the sooner he'll be back for breakfast. He's not convinced and for the first few hundred yards he's in mooch mode. But he perks up when he spots a rabbit and sets off up the lane in a cloud of dust. Parp parp. Road Runner.

I see four hares in a nearby field; as we get nearer they all flatten their ears in unison and amble away across the field, not greatly stressed by our disturbing their breakfast. Cruelly, seeing four hares reminds me of my brother and his follicle shortage! Best not tell him that little nugget.

We pass a familiar farm on the left that appears to have had its defenses breached because a couple of sheep are wandering around between their cars. Sheep are prolific poopers so it's best to keep them away from where you're likely to tread. We crest a rise where we get a view of our goal. Horror of horrors – a van! It's parked right on my spot. It's silhouetted on the skyline and couldn't be more obvious if it tried. We lose sight of it as we dip down and cross the concrete bridge over the beck, but as we rise again, past the sheep-mauled salt bins, there it is. I wasn't dreaming. And now the van has been joined by a man who is fiddling with a rucksack. He's concentrating, pretending to ignore the fact that he's trespassing on my patch. Mind you, he looks as surprised as me as we clamber up towards him wheezing and spluttering.

By now it's nearly 6.00 AM and we look at each other warily as the dog and I approach. The chap is wearing big boots, which is not good; the dog for historical reasons doesn't like people wearing boots. We assume he was kicked before being dumped in the rescue center in France all those years ago. His trauma is buried deep, poor lad. Anyhow, I pop him on the lead and me and the chap introduce ourselves. I have to be frank; I was pretty miffed at having my private spot invaded and I'd already decided to title this segment of my story, 'The Inconsiderate Appearance of Muddy Van Man.'

I'd lined up a mock insult but he took the wind out of my sails by offering a friendly greeting. I'd presumed he was just setting off on a walk but it turns out he had just got back. He'd spent the night in his tent up on the tops, high up to the west. It's a peak I've studied each time I've seen it and have been trying to pluck up courage to tackle it, or at least part way. I'd decided to wait until I've befriended a paramedic who can come with me.

My new friend looks the rustic type. Maybe he is, but during our conversation he tells me he's an architectural consultant in Ambleside, deep in the heart of the Lake District. He's been very busy with city people who have 'more money than space' buying whatever pile of Lakeland stone comes to market.

As we chat I'm feeling more and more of a plonker. Initially I thought he'd encroached on me but, as I find out about more about him, I realize it's me who's intruding. His mother is from Ravenstonedale, 2 miles to the north. His father is from a farm half a mile to the south and he has been living in the area for fifty years, his whole life. He has moved a little further afield now, Sedbergh in fact, all of twelve miles away. He tells me he runs a half marathon from home to Kirkby Stephen to the chippy! He doesn't run home, he tells me, but gets a lift so his dinner doesn't congeal.

He's been camping up on Harter Fell for 'as long as I can remember,' a place he visits to chill out. The view from the top, he tells me, is stunning. If he'd realized I couldn't (at least in my mind) get up there, I could have accused him of being spiteful, but he wasn't - he was a thoroughly decent bloke. It also turned out he knew my hometown of Littleborough, where he had played rugby at the local club up near the lake. That's place I pass regularly on my local cycle rides.

The upshot is that it's me who should slope away and leave him and his dirty van in peace, in his territory where he has spent all his life with his friends and family. The dog has made friends and we say goodbye and head off back. A curlew sings farewell, but it's a slightly unfamiliar song. It's as if the youngsters are learning their trade and haven't yet mastered the familiar rippling trill (I love that expression). Maybe it's not a bloody curlew at all! Dear oh dear, I've a lot to learn.

As we walk down the hill this final time the vista is diminished a little with every step. The distant fells are gradually hidden behind those close by. And though what's close by is lovely, I prefer the full panorama. Right up on the tops the light is brighter, the air cleaner and the silence bigger. Time goes quickly as I daydream and subconsciously soak it all up. The blink of an eye becomes the blink of an hour. In addition, right on the tops, my idiotic ramblings set off on the breeze and keep going; there's nothing to stop them. Lower down they bounce back to make me realize what an uncoordinated jumble I make of things.

* * *

When we arrived for this visit it had rained and rained. For the first day or two the fells were sodden as the spongy moss was overwhelmed. Even the birds hunkered down. Water oozed out, hurried away by temporary new streams. Over a day or two, these gradually slowed and became a trickle, then disappeared altogether. It's dried out now pretty much, enough for my friend to be out camping anyway.

Jan took the dog for a lunchtime potter and came back with a smile on her face. She told me she'd been playing 'statues' with a pair of sheep. She could hear them following her and the dog up the road, but when she turned they stood stock still and stared at her, as if to say, 'Me, following you? Never.' And then again...

I've said before that we create tomorrow's memories today. I think we've accomplished that most days this trip.

Yesterday morning I'd given Richard a lift to Keld, half an hour east. He'd had a night at home because the scheduled stop on his Coast to Coast walk was near enough to allow him a night in his own bed. It was an amazing drive over some of the remotest moorland, on the way passing a sign to Ravenseat, home to 'Our Yorkshire Farm' with Amanda, Clive and their huge tribe. It's a wonderful if remote place to live.

As we drive away there's time for one last curio. Not long after we join the tarmac ribbon we encounter a man standing in the middle of the road. We stop because the alternative is running him down. I wonder if he's in some sort of trouble. I wind the window down and ask him if he's OK, to which he replies, in a pronounced east London accent, 'Nice again, isn't it? I love it up here.'

We chat for a few minutes and learn he's lived a couple of miles away for a few years, having retired up here from London. He didn't want anything and he was in good health, so the only thing we could think was that he was desperate for a chat! That was all fine with us, and it's no problem up here in the wilderness; but if he'd tried to flag a car down for a natter where we live he'd have got an earful of fruity language, or mown down.

The End (officially)

There's the introduction without which you've probably managed perfectly
well so far.
But it follows, so if you must......

40

The Vault - Beginning at the End...

This bit may give some context as to why I'm keen to keep moving. The end of our boating years saw us return to land to be with family; in particular, two new grandsons and one poorly brother. Six years on, the youngsters have moved away with their mum and dad and Jan's sibling has died.

We miss them all, of course we do. Ian suffered ill health for many years and reached the point where he'd had enough. We believe he chose the moment to leave us. So, now we look back to a time when he was well, back to childhood when his innocent smile shone from photographs. These were the years when things were carefree and fun. Two generations down the line, those innocent, wonderful years are the ones our grandsons are living in their new home in the Cumbrian Fells. Their mum and dad have created a platform for an incredible upbringing. When they look back in the future I hope they see a shining sun. They are only an hour and a half away so we can pop up and share their new life from time to time.

So that's the past and present, and right now Jan and I have a void. Worse, we're faced with the prospect of predictability and sameness, neither of which we cope with very well. We like where we live - nice house, nice people - but it's the thought that when we park the car on the drive, we've hit the buffers. That there's no way forward. What we need instead of a terminus is a crossroads so we can at least have the opportunity for exploration. Invariably we'll come back home, but we need the option to take one of these roads and just keep going, have a new adventure.

Jan said to me a few months ago that she didn't want to move again. She is happy where she is - friends, familiar shops, good health care. etc. Of course, we are getting on a bit and we do need to be sensible as far as the twilight years are concerned, but Jan's words sent a bit of a shiver through me. They implied a finality that we've never had before. We've always had something to take us forward. Watching Bargain Hunt on daytime TV is OK every now and then, but for ever?

The boat was comfortable, safe and warm, but what made it special was the excitement of the next bend. I look back and see in my mind's eye two aspects of this. One, the anticipation of finding out what's round the corner. Two, making the most out of where we are before we move on, because going round the next bend can't be undone. What's behind are memories, things that will enliven our rocking-chair years - which will come soon enough.

We boated for twelve years on the waterways of the UK and Europe. We visited some remarkable places and met some wonderful people. So, how could we top something like that? The fact is we can't. We haven't even tried. In the six years since we ended boating years we have had some great times with family and we've worked hard. But it's time to look beyond the garden fence. Jan has subsequently changed her mind about staying put for definite and is open to change. Not change for change's sake, but if the right opportunity comes along at least we can have a good look. We can take the blinkers off. New adventures are born with an idea. The trick is to recognize that idea and be willing to run with it. Most ideas fizzled out but boating life didn't. We need to find something else that develops and keeps us out of the armchair.

But, in 2011, ten years ago as I write, I noticed increasing discomfort in my legs and back. I was aching like mad after only a few hundred yards where previously I'd do anything up to thirty miles without much of a problem. It came on gradually over a few weeks. I sort of knew there was something amiss, but convinced myself I was OK. Eventually I couldn't ignore it and it got to the point where I all but gave up cycling. It wasn't until 2015 that I was diagnosed with type 2 diabetes but, more worryingly, a blocked aorta where it meets the iliac leg arteries (caused by smoking). Bit of a blow this. It was either a big (and risky) operation or try a change of lifestyle, including diet and exercise regime, to try and create new blood vessels; in effect, to get blood down south. *'Then we'll see how you go,'* said the surgeon. Which was better than, *'I'll see you Monday for an op.'* I was frightened enough to really follow doctor's orders. In fact, since that moment, I've believed if you're frightened enough and get your head in gear you can change just about anything.

So, I began a strict low carbohydrate diet which would control the T2 diabetes. Additionally, the lack of surplus glucose in the blood would help with the circulation. Excess glucose is inflammatory, which is bad for the blood vessels. I began to walk and walk. Over the space of a year I went from pottering one mile a day to ten. Whereas I used to be in pain after a couple of hundred meters, I could now cope with a lot more. I'd go ten times around a circuit near my home. In one year I walked the equivalent of Lancashire to Barcelona and back. But eventually, I got a bit bored of Barcelona. Plus, all the walking began to take a toll on my hips.

So, an alternative form of exercise was needed ... think bike. It was with a spring in my step (and a bit of trepidation) that I borrowed my stepdaughter's mountain bike. It didn't go too well, in all honesty. On my first ride for about five years, I was overtaken by a jogger. Things did improve somewhat but I was nowhere near as capable as I used to be, despite all the walking.

Then, one day, I saw chap on an electric bike. I was struggling to walk up a steep hill when he zoomed past, apparently effortlessly. To be honest, that moment changed my whole outlook. I researched and bought one. With all the peripherals (drinks bottle, luminous clothing, etc.) it was pretty expensive (for me, anyway), but it gave me a new lease of life. In fact at this point, our car, which I'd used as a workhorse while renovating five houses in as many years, was on its last legs and my new bike was actually worth ten times the car!

So, having ridden my e-bike for a while, I have now been inspired to put pen to paper once again. One man, after he'd read *A Narrowboat at Large*, emailed me through my website. He told me that we were an inspiration, that's me and my wife, Jan. That's a first - I can tell you I've never been called an inspiration before. He has been poorly himself, and his wife had just been diagnosed with Parkinson's. They both walk the canal towpaths in Shropshire to keep as fit as possible. It's where we first lived on a boat and I've written about the area quite extensively, so he could relate my tales to the places he's walked. I've just re-read his message to me and it's brought a tear to my eye. That one email is worth the effort of the hundreds and hundreds of hours I've spent at my computer keyboard trying to arrange lots of words into a semi-coherent tale.

I've also written about my management of my ailments, particularly the diabetes. People have reacted to that, too; in fact, one or two have told me they've had a change of lifestyle as a result, which is great.

My wife overcame cancer twice, against the odds, which was why we took up boating in the first place. We decided to get on with something before it was too late. We were under fifty years old and people asked us how we could afford to do it at our age. My answer was always, *'We can't afford not to do it.'*

Perhaps this book is also for people who may need a nudge to try something fresh or get themselves back on track for whatever reason. As I ride, I remind myself that I'm doing it for a purpose and realize I'm lucky to be enjoying it at the same time. I see joggers (or runners - when does a jog become a run?) who don't look to be enjoying it at all; they look in a world of pain and can't wait to get home for a brew and an egg butty. All I know is that I continue to enjoy getting out and about, whether on bike or in boots.

Glossary

This book may have inadvertently taken it's leave of The British Isles. Because some of the language is English (UK), or more accurately English (Lancashire), I thought I'd better explain one or two words or sayings, words that may not have travelled well.

In addition, if you're American you'll see plenty of words ending ...OUR, whereas you end them....OR. So, do me a favo(u)r and don't mark me down on spelling.

Glossary

Audi – A German motor car. Greeting in Texas.

Blob – Rotund person (me)

By Gum – Goodness me / my words

Chortling – Mixture of laughing and chuckling

Claggy – Stickily clinging, as in mud

Cock a Snook – Openly show contempt for or to defy

Croak – Die / peg-it

Dawdle – Go slowly / lag (more me than scoot)

Derring-do – Bold, daring deeds

Essex – English county where they say innit instead of isn't it.

Billericay – A town in Essex. Innit.

Fit as a fiddle – A healthy, jogging violinist

Flobber – Fat / spare flesh

Git – Often referring to an older person and preceded by an unpleasant adjective

Gloucestershire Old Spots- A rare breed of pig

Gordon Brown - Prime Minister at the time

Gusset - Additional piece of cloth used to strengthen a garment

Hollerin' - shouting

Hooter - Nose

Hurtle - Move at speed (not in my case)

In a huff - In an annoyed state

In a pickle - In trouble

It Ain't Half Hot Mum- UK TV programme. Not PC these days.

Jaunt - Short journey, often taken for pleasure

Jogging bottoms - Item of clothing as opposed to buttocks

Junker - Something ready for scrapping

Knobbly - Irregular in shape

Larder - Food store

Lug - Carry, drag

Lumped - Heaved / lifted

Mooch - Walk slowly without much purpose

Motley - Incongruously varied in appearance (ill-matched clothes)

Murky - Dark / gloomy

Nabbed - Caught

Natty - Smart / clever / fashionable

Niggle - Irritation

Parky - Cold, chilly

Pendragon - Surname of Arthur and Uther of Arthurian legend fame

Piddly - Small

Pillock - Stupid person / something hard to rest your head on

Plonker - A foolish or inept person

Poddling - Moving slowly / ambling

Porky - Overweight and chilly

Portly - Rotund, as in figure

Punter - Customer

Ralphed - Vomited. (Ralph is onomatopoeic)

Rickety - Flimsily built / unsafe

Scoot - Go quickly (not in my case)

Sticks - Countryside / rural area

Stout - Reference drink - Strong dark beer.

Tiddler - Small (as in fish)

Tizz - Excited

Waddle - A walking gait not unlike a duck

West Bromwich Albion- Soccer club, along with Wolves

Whoopin' - random cry or expression of delight

Wombles - A fictional TV characters know for collecting junk

Jo's Books

You can see all Jo's books at: jomay.uk

A Narrowboat at Large is the first of three best-selling books in Jo's **At Large** series that chronicle he and his wife Jan's waterways adventures. When asked by a friend to explain this rash, knuckle-headed decision, Jo said:

'So why did we take to the water? My wife can't swim, the dog hates it and I prefer beer.

The main reason is that my wife's doctors had told her she was in real trouble so we developed a different perspective about the future than many people. We needed to get on with things.

We knew nothing about narrowboats and how we would cope being cooped up together – particularly when it's minus five and the nearest shop is miles away. We had a mountain to climb – which you can only do by using locks – and we'd never done a lock.

A more accurate analogy is shooting the rapids. Our venture took on a life of its own and we were washed down stream on a tide of enthusiasm and ignorance. We had to make it work or the people who had laughed and scoffed that we were mad would be proved right.

Well, make it work we did, and we boated for twelve years – first on narrowboats then an old barge on the continent.

It was marvellous and it possibly saved Jan's life.'

A Barge at Large and A Barge at Large II are light-hearted accounts of what happened when Jo and Jan May bought a 100-year-old Dutch barge and travelled in Holland, Belgium and France. In the beginning the engine barely ran, the heating system didn't work and the rusty patches were growing like fungus on an old loaf.

With professional help generally unaffordable they learned to do things themselves, including kicking numerous bits of misbehaving equipment in an attempt to make them see reason. Gradually, things improved to the point where they could at least have lunch without an alarm going off.

Traveling from the north of Holland, through Belgium to Burgundy in France, they had less space, but more freedom and had less cash but were immeasurably richer. There was no keeping up with the Jones' – if anyone started being pompous they could untie the ropes and go elsewhere to experience the pleasures and quirks of new countries and a wacky assortment of people who'd also drifted into a watery existence from any number of directions.

A wonderful life where they endured misbehaving lavatories and dribbly windows, but also the delights of wildlife, windmills and wine.

Fiction

Operation Vegetable

Deep in the English countryside is Watergrove marina, home to a group of unlikely characters living on their narrowboats.

Life is carefree until a local land-owner decides he wants to build three luxury houses on the resident's vegetable plot.

Step forward Judy, a lady of physical substance, fierce determination and jocular disposition, who leads our ageing boaters in a counter-offensive code-named 'Operation Vegetable'.

H.Q. is the local pub and it's here that our ageing boaters raise a creaking battalion.

The boaters find help from an ageing rock star and a TV Gardening programme. Skirmish follows skirmish until one of the boaters is severely injured and the stakes are raised.

Has the despotic land-owner, a man of few morals, driven by power and greed, finally met his match?

Can the boaters overcome this scourge - or have they simply lost the plot?

Flawed Liaisons

Harry Dunn is an ordinary man living an ordinary life. But a series of events turn his world upside down. His life implodes and he is forced to run.

He is on the ragged edge when a surprise inheritance offers him a lifeline. But it's a poisoned chalice.

He hides away in the underbelly of a prosperous market town among the destitute where he befriends Mary, a woman tormented by her own demons.

Both are forced to confront their pasts as they try to unravel the mystery at the heart of Harry's downfall. What they discover is evil from the past that refuses to die - depravity carried through time in black hearts.

Harry and Mary forge a bond, a liaison born from the misery of their pasts. They have both suffered but find that others have paid a far higher price.

COMING SOON

Twice Removed

In a quirky town nestled in the Northumbrian hills lives Tony Mason.

He's a watcher of people. Jokingly referred to as a snoop, by the landlady of The Bull public house, where Tony and his wacky assortment of friends gather.

The town is called Thistledean, a unique blend of the recent past and distant past, held together by inhabitants determined to protect the life they used to have and seem to still enjoy.

Tony befriends a special old lady, a visitor on a 'pensioners special' coach outing. He catches her as she stumbles while getting off a bus. A simple encounter but the start of a wonderful friendship. She is a determined character with a jumbled past who welcomes Tony's support as she tries to find out who she is.

Thistledean is a peculiar place but a warm place. As one transient visitor said, 'It's somewhere I'm not sure I want to visit again, but perversely a place I would like to live.'

About the Author

Jo lives in Lancashire with wife Jan and dog Tache.

He began writing monthly articles for a canal magazine in 2007. Catastrophically (for the magazine!) following an 'editorial misunderstanding', they parted company. Jo began to chronicle their travels which ultimately resulted in his three best-selling 'At Large' books beginning with A Narrowboat at Large. Jo describes their memories as a huge warm cloud in which he and Jan can wallow during long winter evenings and in their rocking-chair years. Magical times.

After destroying the UK's canal infrastructure on two Narrowboats and rearranging a fair amount of continental waterways heritage on a rusty old Dutch Barge, their boating days came to an end in 2015, to everyone's relief except theirs.

Boating days behind him, Jo's new challenge is an e-bike. However, to mix metaphors, it's not all been plain sailing. Ordeals on Wheels sums it up quite nicely.

You can connect with me on:

 https://jomay.uk

 https://www.facebook.com/JoMayWriter/?ref=bookmarks

Printed in Great Britain
by Amazon

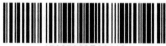